PreTest®

Genetics

Notice

Medicine is an ever-changing science. As new research and clinical experience broaden our knowledge, changes in treatment and drug therapy are required. The authors and the publisher of this work have checked with sources believed to be reliable in their efforts to provide information that is complete and generally in accord with the standards accepted at the time of publication. However, in view of the possibility of human error or changes in medical sciences, neither the authors nor the publisher nor any other party who has been involved in the preparation or publication of this work warrants that the information contained herein is in every respect accurate or complete, and they are not responsible for any errors or omissions or for the results obtained from use of such information. Readers are encouraged to confirm the information contained herein with other sources. For example and in particular, readers are advised to check the product information sheet included in the package of each drug they plan to administer to be certain that the information contained in this book is accurate and that changes have not been made in the recommended dose or in the contraindications for administration. This recommendation is of particular importance in connection with new or infrequently used drugs.

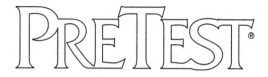

Genetics

PreTest®
Self-Assessment
and Review

Second Edition

Janice Finkelstein, M.D.
Assistant Professor of Pediatrics
The Johns Hopkins University School of Medicine
Baltimore, Maryland

Golder Wilson, M.D., Ph.D.
Professor of Pediatrics
The University of Texas Southwestern Medical School
Dallas, Texas

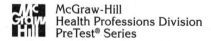 McGraw-Hill
Health Professions Division
PreTest® Series

New York   St. Louis   San Francisco   Auckland
Bogotá   Caracas   Lisbon   London   Madrid
Mexico City   Milan   Montreal   New Delhi
San Juan   Singapore   Sydney   Tokyo   Toronto

McGraw-Hill

*A Division of The **McGraw·Hill** Companies*

1 2 3 4 5 6 7 8 9 0 DOCDOC 9 9 8 7 6 5

ISBN 0-07-052083-6

The editors were Gail Gavert and Bruce MacGregor.
The production supervisor was Gyl A. Favours.
This book was set in Times Roman by Compset, Inc.
R.R. Donnelley & Sons was printer and binder.

Library of Congress Cataloging-in-Publication Data
Genetics : PreTest self-assessment and review /
   Janice Finkelstein, Golder Wilson. — 2nd ed.
      p. cm.
   Includes bibliographical references.
   ISBN 0-07-052083-6
   1. Medical genetics—Examinations, questions, etc. 2. Human
genetics—Examinations, questions, etc. I. Finkelstein, Janice.
II. Wilson, Golder.
   [DNLM: 1. Genetics, Medical—examination questions.   QZ 18.2 G328
1996]
RB155.G395 1996
616'.042'076—dc20
DNLM/DLC
for Library of Congress   95-4139

Contents

Introduction

Each *PreTest® Self-Assessment and Review* allows medical students to comprehensively and conveniently assess and review their knowledge of a particular basic science, in this instance Genetics. The 500 questions parallel the format and degree of difficulty of the questions found in the United States Medical Licensing Examination (USMLE) Step 1. Practicing physicians who want to hone their skills before USMLE Step 3 or recertification may find this to be a good beginning in their review process.

Each question is accompanied by an answer, a paragraph explanation, and a specific page reference to an appropriate textbook or journal article. A bibliography listing sources can be found following the last chapter of this text.

An effective way to use this PreTest is to allow yourself one minute to answer each question in a given chapter. As you proceed, indicate your answer beside each question. By following this suggestion, you approximate the time limits imposed by the Step.

After you finish going through the questions in the section, spend as much time as you need verifying your answers and carefully reading the explanations provided. Pay special attention to the explanations for the questions you answered incorrectly—but read *every* explanation. The authors of this material have designed the explanations to reinforce and supplement the information tested by the questions. If you feel you need further information about the material covered, consult and study the references indicated.

PreTest®

Genetics

Basic Genetics

DIRECTIONS: Each question below contains five suggested responses. Select the **one best** response to each question.

1. The age of onset of a degenerative neurologic disease is 35. Epidemiologic study of affected persons indicates that most cases occur in the spring, are isolated (i.e., no neighbors or relatives are affected) and occur equally in men and women. However, a subset of cases consists of two affected siblings in a family. The best description of this disease is

(A) inherited
(B) genetic
(C) sporadic
(D) congenital
(E) familial

2. If a DNA fingerprinting study indicates that a pair of twins are identical at all five loci examined, then these twins are best described as

(A) monozygous
(B) concordant
(C) discordant
(D) dizygous
(E) conjoint

3. What is the baseline risk for congenital malformations in the average pregnancy?

(A) 2/10,000
(B) 2/1000
(C) 2/100
(D) 2/10
(E) 2/5

4. A man and a woman who both have Bb genotypes at a locus will produce zygotes in which of the following ratios?

(A) 1BB:1Bb:1bb
(B) 2BB:1Bb:1bb
(C) 1BB:2Bb:1bb
(D) 1BB:2Bb:2bb
(E) 1BB:3Bb

5. What proportion of families with three children will have all boys?

(A) 1/3
(B) 1/6
(C) 1/8
(D) 1/12
(E) 1/64

Questions 6–10

A man and his wife who have two children, the second of whom has a genetic disorder, came to the physician's office. They are currently expecting another child. The physician obtains the pedigree shown below. It is assumed that the genetic disorder of the second child is not the result of a new mutation.

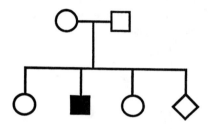

6. Assuming that the genetic disorder in question is X-linked, what is the most likely genetic status of the mother and the affected child?

(A) Homozygote (mother); heterozygote (affected child)
(B) Heterozygote (mother); hemizygote (affected child)
(C) Hemizygote (mother); homozygote (affected child)
(D) Autozygote (mother); hemizygote (affected child)
(E) Unable to determine from information given

7. Assuming X-linked inheritance, what are the chances that the fetus is an unaffected carrier?

(A) 2/3
(B) 1/2
(C) 1/3
(D) 1/4
(E) Indeterminable

8. Now assume that the genetic disorder in question is inherited in an autosomal recessive fashion. What is the most likely genetic status of the mother, father, and affected child?

(A) Homozygote (mother); homozygote (father); heterozygote (affected child)
(B) Heterozygote (mother); heterozygote (father); homozygote (affected child)
(C) Hemizygote (mother); homozygote (father); autozygote (affected child)
(D) Autozygote (mother); hemizygote (father); hemizygote (affected child)
(E) Unable to determine from information given

9. Assuming autosomal recessive inheritance, what are the chances that the fetus is affected?

(A) 2/3
(B) 1/2
(C) 1/3
(D) 1/4
(E) Unable to determine from information given

10. Assuming autosomal recessive inheritance, what are the chances that the eldest unaffected daughter is a carrier?

(A) 2/3
(B) 1/2
(C) 1/3
(D) 1/4
(E) Unable to determine from information given

11. A man and woman who both have Bb genotypes at a locus will produce what proportion of bb children?

(A) 100 percent
(B) 75 percent
(C) 50 percent
(D) 25 percent
(E) 0 percent

12. The average incidence of common single malformations such as cleft palate or spina bifida is

(A) 1/10,000
(B) 1/5000
(C) 1/1000
(D) 1/500
(E) 1/100

13. The term *reverse genetics* refers to the

(A) identification of genes based on position alone
(B) identification of genes based on the biochemical features of the disease
(C) study of X-linked disorders
(D) study of non-Mendelian patterns of inheritance
(E) study of clinical genetic disorders

DIRECTIONS: Each numbered question or incomplete statement below is
NEGATIVELY phrased. Select the **one best** lettered response.

14. Mendel's laws apply to every statement below EXCEPT

(A) many traits are determined by a pair of hereditary units (i.e., *genes* or *alleles*)
(B) gametes (i.e., ova or sperm) each receive one of the paired alleles
(C) there is random sorting of alleles into ova and sperm
(D) alleles at loci on the same chromosome may segregate together
(E) the pair of alleles is reconstituted by zygote formation

15. All the following statements regarding single-gene defects are true EXCEPT

(A) they are inherited in a Mendelian fashion
(B) they are caused by mutant genes
(C) over 4000 disorders are known
(D) the biochemical defect is known in less than 100 disorders
(E) most defects are rare

DIRECTIONS: Each group of questions below consists of lettered headings followed by a set of numbered items. For each numbered item select the **one** lettered heading with which it is **most** closely associated. Each lettered heading may be used **once, more than once or not at all.**

Questions 16–17

Match each term listed below with the appropriate definition.

(A) Cosegregation of alleles
(B) One phenotype, multiple genotypes
(C) Nonrandom allele association
(D) One locus, multiple mutant alleles
(E) One locus, multiple normal alleles

16. Polymorphism

17. Linkage disequilibrium

Questions 18–19

Match each term that follows with the phrase that best defines it.

(A) A region of DNA encoding RNA
(B) Alternative form of a gene
(C) Complete set of genes in cell or organism
(D) Abnormal gene
(E) Position of gene on chromosome

18. Allele

19. Locus

Questions 20–21

Match each genetic disease category with the phrase that best defines it.

(A) Mendelian inheritance
(B) Human cancers
(C) Most common type of human genetic disease
(D) Major cause of miscarriages
(E) Maternally derived

20. Chromosomal disorders

21. Multifactorial disorders

Questions 22–24

Match the number of possible alleles at a single locus with the number of genotypes that could result.

(A) Three possible genotypes
(B) Six possible genotypes
(C) Nine possible genotypes
(D) Ten possible genotypes
(E) Sixteen possible genotypes

22. Two alleles

23. Three alleles

24. Four alleles

Questions 25–27

For each family history listed below, select the pedigree that most accurately represents it.

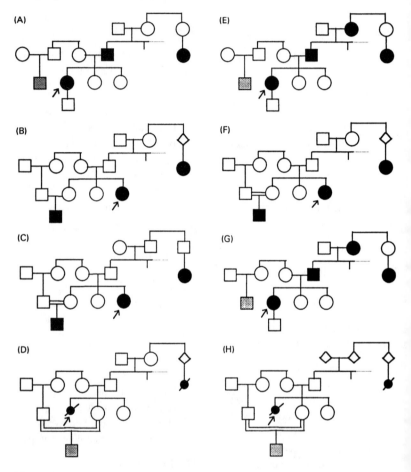

25. A couple has three girls, the last of whom is affected with cystic fibrosis. The first-born daughter married her first cousin—that is, the son of her mother's sister, and they have a son with cystic fibrosis. The father has a female cousin with cystic fibrosis on his mother's side.

26. A couple learns that their first-born daughter, one of three girls, has neurofibromatosis. The father learns that he too is affected after his physician recognizes café au lait spots and neurofibromas. After discussing his family history, the father realizes that his mother is affected, as is a daughter of his mother's sister. His wife recalls that she has a brother whose son has cystic fibrosis. The daughter with neurofibromatosis has a normal son.

27. A young couple has two living daughters; the first pregnancy was a stillborn female who was affected with achondroplasia. The first-born daughter married her first cousin—that is, the son of her mother's sister. This consanguineous couple had a son with phenylketonuria (PKU). The father has a female first cousin who was also stillborn with features of achondroplastic dwarfism.

Questions 28–29

Match each of the following descriptions with the correct pedigree symbol.

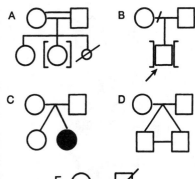

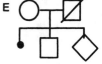

28. Discordant twins

29. Divorced couple with child adopted out

Questions 30–31

For each genetic disease category listed below, select the approximate incidence figures most likely to be associated with it.

(A) 0.3 to 0.4 percent
(B) 0.5 to 0.7 percent
(C) 3 to 5 percent
(D) 10 to 25 percent
(E) 50 percent

30. Chromosomal disorders at birth

31. Genetic disorders that necessitate admission to a pediatric hospital

Questions 32–36

   Diane and David, recently engaged, consult a physician about their risk of having a child with absent fingers (ectrodactyly). David's family history is normal, but Diane has several relatives with ectrodactyly. Diane has one sibling, a brother, with absent fingers. Her father is an only child. Diane's mother, Paula, has normal hands. Paula was the first-born child in her family, followed by a brother, a sister, and a brother. Paula's father Ronald, the youngest of his siblings, had ectrodactyly. Ronald's oldest brothers, both with absent fingers, were identical twins. Next, in order of age, was a normal sister, a brother with absent fingers who was put up for adoption, and another normal sister. Ronald's elder sister had two normal daughters. Ronald's parents, both deceased, were thought to be normal. Paula's maternal grandparents were also deceased; her mother had a younger brother John. John's only daughter married Paula's youngest brother, and they have a normal son.

   For each family member listed below, select the pedigree symbol that most aptly describes him or her. You will have to construct your own pedigree based on the case history to answer this question.

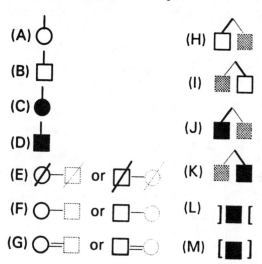

32. Individual I-2

33. Individual II-1

34. Individual II-5

35. Individual III-8

36. Individual IV-3

Questions 37–46

Match each of the following descriptions with the correct pedigree symbol.

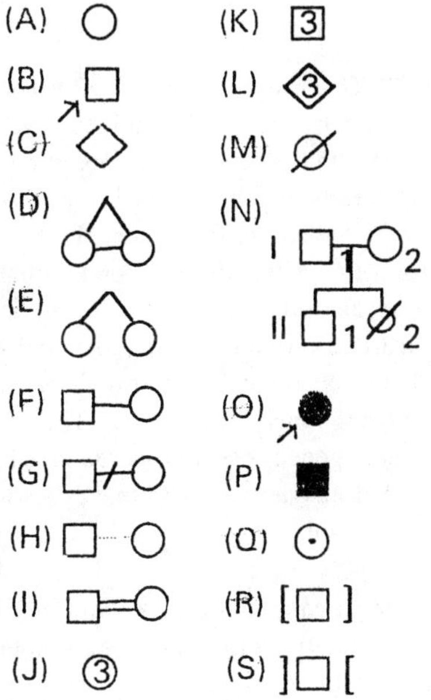

(A) ◯

(B) ◻

(C) ◇

(D) △◯ (with connecting line)

(E) (linked symbols)

(F) ◻—◯

(G) ◻⫻◯

(H) ◻⋯◯

(I) ◻═◯

(J) ③

(K) ③ (boxed)

(L) ◇③

(M) ⊘

(N)
I   ◻₁—◯₂
II   ◻₁ ⊘₂

(O) ● (with arrow)

(P) ■

(Q) ⊙

(R) [◻]

(S)] ◻ [

37. Unaffected individual sex unspecified

38. Unaffected female, deceased

39. Affected female proband

40. Adopted into family

41. Female carrier

42. Monozygotic twins

43. Consanguineous marriage

44. Union

45. Divorce

46. Prenatal death

Basic Genetics
Answers

1.   The answer is E. *(Gelehrter, pp 27–29. Thompson, 5/e, pp 53–59.)* The term *familial* indicates that a trait or disorder tends to cluster in families. A *genetic* disorder is one in which there is evidence that a gene or chromosome is involved in the susceptibility to the disease. Evidence for vertical transmission (e.g., father to daughter) is necessary for a disorder to be labeled *inherited*. *Sporadic* indicates that evidence for vertical transmission or familial clustering is lacking. *Congenital* simply means present at birth. Note that many congenital diseases (e.g., congenital AIDS) are not genetic, that adult-onset diseases may be genetic without being congenital, and that diseases may be familial (e.g., chickenpox) without being inherited or genetic. The eugenics movement was based on a fallacy about genetics as it proposed breeding restrictions based on the assumption that all genetic traits (e.g., Down syndrome) would have a high risk for transmission.

2.   The answer is A. *(Gelehrter, p 60.)* Identical patterns of polymorphic alleles at five separate loci imply that the twins derived from the same zygote (*monozygous* or identical twins). Splitting of the embryo may occur early (single amnion and placenta—diamnionic monozygotic twins) or later (two amnions and one or two placentas—diamniotic, mono-, or dichorionic twins). Early splitting of a portion of the embryo produces *conjoint* twins that are fused together (Siamese twins). Double ovulation is one mechanism that causes two separate zygotes to implant in the same uterus (*dizygous* or fraternal twins). Such twins will always have two amnions but may have fused placentas that make them difficult to distinguish from monozygotic twins. *Concordant* versus *discordant* twins indicates whether they share or do not share a particular trait. Twin studies are enormously important in revealing the genetic etiology of complex traits.

3.   The answer is C. *(Gelehrter, pp 27–30. Thompson, 5/e, p 2.)* The incidence of major congenital anomalies or genetic disease at birth is at least 2 to 3 percent of all pregnancies. If children are followed until age 7, the rate approaches 10 percent due to a variety of problems, such as hearing and heart defects, that are not appreciated early. Genetic disorders affect every organ system and cause a significant portion of infant mortality.

4. **The answer is C.** *(Gelehrter, pp 27–30. Thompson, 5/e, p 2.)* Possible combinations of alleles in gametes form the basis of most genetic risk calculations and can be simplified by using the Punnett square below.

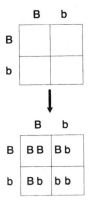

The parental alleles are aligned on each side of the square, and the potential combinations of gametes are listed in each compartment. Ratios of the genotypes can then be read directly.

5. **The answer is C.** *(Gelehrter, pp 30–31. Thompson, 5/e, pp 146–147.)* Each pregnancy may be taken as an independent event with a 1/2 chance of male offspring. Therefore, the chance that three separate pregnancies will result in the birth of a male child is $1/2 \times 1/2 \times 1/2$ or 1/8.

6–10. **The answers are: 6-B, 7-D, 8-B, 9-D, 10-A.** *(Gelehrter, pp 27– 45. Thompson, 5/e, pp 53–82.)* The genetic status or genotype of an individual is determined by the two alleles, which are located on the two homologous chromosomes. *Homozygotes* have identical alleles on the two chromosomes, whereas *heterozygotes* have two different alleles. *Autozygotes* are homozygous individuals in whom the alleles are identical on the basis of consanguinity or unusual chromosome segregation. Generally, heterozygotes have one normal allele and one mutant allele. However, the term is also used when there are two different normal alleles. A *compound heterozygote* refers to an individual with two different mutant alleles. When referring to X-linked disorders, it must be remembered that, whereas women have two homologous X chromosomes, men have one X and one Y chromosome and, therefore, only one X-linked allele. They are referred to as *hemizygotes*.

When evaluating an X-linked pedigree, it must be remembered that a man inherits his X chromosome from his mother, who is, therefore, a carrier for the abnormal allele. In a recessive pedigree, the affected individual must have two abnormal copies of the gene in question, one inherited from each unaffected, heterozygous, carrier parent.

The genotype of the heterozygous parents in question may be denoted as $a^1 a^2$ where a^1 is the normal allele and a^2 is the mutant allele. The ratios of possible combinations of alleles in gametes is $1a^1 a^1 : 2a^1 a^2 : 1a^2$. When the clinical status of the individual is unknown, as in the case of the unborn fetus, the chances are 1/4 that the individual is affected and 2/4 or 1/2 that the individual is a heterozygote. However, when it is known that the individual is unaffected, there are only three possible combinations of parental alleles. The individual has a 1/3 chance of being homozygous unaffected and a 2/3 chance of being heterozygous based on the two different parental combinations of alleles (a^1 from mother/a^2 from father or a^2 from mother/a^1 from father).

11. The answer is D. *(Gelehrter, pp 27–30.)* For each parent, 50 percent of the gametes (i.e., eggs and sperm) will have a B allele, and 50 percent will have a b allele. The distribution of alleles in zygotes can be derived using the Punnett square below.

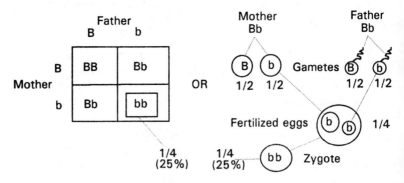

The bb genotype in offspring, highlighted in the figure, accounts for 1/4 or 25 percent of the possibilities. Alternatively, one can calculate a 1/2 probability for a b allele from the mother, a 1/2 probability of a b allele from the father, and a joint probability of $1/2 \times 1/2 = 1/4$ for the bb genotype in a zygote.

12. The answer is C. *(Gelehrter, pp 27–30. Thompson, 5/e, p 2.)* Common birth defects have an incidence of about 1/1000 live births. Examples include neural tube defects (i.e., spina bifida/myelomeningocele), most congenital heart defects, isolated cleft palate and cleft lip with cleft palate, congenital dislocated hip, and hydrocephalus. Precise incidence figures vary by defect and population. While a 1/1000 incidence may not seem "common," this translates to 300 cases per year in a state such as Texas (300,000 annual births) and 3000 cases per year in the United States (3 million annual births).

13. The answer is A. *(Gelehrter, pp 193–207. Thompson, 5/e, pp 167–199.)* The term *reverse genetics,* also known as positional cloning, refers to the identification and cloning of a gene based on its position alone. This allows for the identification of genes whose biochemical function is unknown. Once the gene is identified and characterized, mutations may be analyzed, and the nature of the protein product may be identified. This, in turn, allows for a better understanding of the cause of disease. Many different molecular methods have been used in the physical mapping and subsequent cloning of genes, including somatic cell genetics, in situ hybridization, and genetic linkage analysis.

14. The answer is D. *(Gelehrter, pp 27–28. Thompson, 5/e, p 2.)* Mendel's laws assert that (1) traits reflect the inheritance of units subsequently called *genes,* (2) genes come in pairs that separate into different gametes at meiosis *(segregation)*, and (3) gene pairs segregate independently of one another. Cosegregation of synthetic alleles (i.e., alleles on the same chromosome) violates Mendel's law of independent assortment, although it represents the phenomenon of genetic linkage. Mendel's pea loci were on different chromosomes and, thus, were inherited independently. Recently discovered inheritance mechanisms that violate Mendel's laws include genomic imprinting, mitochondrial inheritance, and germinal mosaicism.

15. The answer is D. *(Gelehrter, pp 27–44. Thompson, 5/e, pp 53–95.)* Single-gene disorders are caused by mutations that have a major effect on the patient's medical condition. They are inherited in simple Mendelian fashion. Over 4000 disorders are known. These disorders are catalogued both on line and in hard copy in *Mendelian Inheritance in Man* edited by Dr. Victor McKusick. The biochemical defect is known in several hundred of these disorders. Although individually rare, when taken together, single-gene disorders account for a significant percentage of morbidity and mortality, especially in children.

16–17. The answers are: 16-E, 17-C. *(Gelehrter, pp 299–311. Thompson, 5/e, pp 115–125.)* Polymorphic loci have multiple alleles because of DNA sequence variation. The DNA sequence changes may involve restriction sites (i.e., restriction fragment length polymorphisms, RFLPs), repeated segments (i.e., variable number of tandem repeats, VNTRs), or expressed regions (i.e., protein polymorphisms). Polymorphisms allow deduction of relationships between loci (i.e., cosegregation or linkage of particular alleles in a family) and between alleles (i.e., disequilibrium of allele with allele or allele with disease). Different mutant alleles may cause indistinguishable phenotypes (allelic heterogeneity) as may mutations at different loci (genetic heterogeneity).

18–19. The answers are: 18-B, 19-E. *(Gelehrter, pp 27–29. Thompson, 5/e, pp 427–442.)* Each organism is defined by a characteristic number and arrangement of DNA sequences—that is, the *genome. Genes* are the basic units of this hereditary material, and pairs or combinations of genes act to determine traits. In modern terms, genes are segments of DNA encoding RNA molecules that are used for cell structure or protein translation. Because mutations constantly change DNA sequences, different versions of genes arise. Each gene occupies a particular position on a chromosome (*locus*); variant genes that occupy the same chromosomal locus are termed *alleles.* Alleles are not necessarily abnormal, since many mutations do not alter protein function. Loci with many alleles are called *polymorphic,* and these variant alleles are useful as genetic markers in family studies.

20–21. The answers are: 20-D, 21-C. *(Gelehrter, pp 3–5. Thompson, 5/e, pp 4–7.)* Genetic disorders may be classified in several major categories. Chromosomal disorders are caused by the deletion or duplication of either pieces of chromosomes or entire chromosomes and are a common cause of miscarriage. Single-gene disorders, also known as Mendelian disorders, are due to defects in single genes. Multifactorial disorders, the most common type of human genetic disease, represent the composite effects of multiple genes, each of which contributes a minor component to the disorder. Environmental factors also play a role in multifactorial disorders. Many common diseases, such as coronary artery disease or diabetes mellitus, are multifactorial disorders. In human cancers, malignancy may result from a mutation in a gene involved in the regulation of cell growth. These mutations occur in specific somatic cells rather than in all cells of the body. Defects in mitochondrial DNA may also result in disease. Since mitochondria are cytoplasmic organelles inherited via the cytoplasm of the ovum, these disorders are always maternally inherited.

22–24. The answers are: 22-A, 23-B, 24-D. *(Gelehrter, pp 49–52. Thompson, 5/e, p 179.)* For a two-allele system (e.g., A and B), three genotypes are possible (i.e., AA, AB, and BB). In a three-allele system (e.g., A, B, and C), six genotypes are possible (i.e., AA, AB, AC, BB, BC, and CC). For a four-allele system, there are ten possible genotypes (i.e., AA, AB, AC, AD, BB, BC, BD, CC, CD, and DD). In general, if a is the number of alleles, a is also the number of homozygotes and $a(a - 1)/2$ is the number of heterozygotes. The total number of genotypes is the sum of homozygotes and heterozygotes or $a + a(a - 1)/2 = (a + a^2)/2$.

25–27. The answers are: 25-F, 26-E, 27-H. *(Gelehrter, pp 27–29. Thompson, 5/e, pp 53–57.)* It is important that the pedigree be an accurate reflection of the family history and that information is not recorded unless specifically mentioned. For question 25, pedigree (B) omits the double line needed to indicate consanguinity, and pedigree (C) assumes that the father's affected cousin is the offspring of his uncle rather than being unspecified. For question 26, pedigree (A) does not show the father's mother as being affected, and pedigree (G) shows his nephew as being the offspring of his sister rather than his brother. For question 27, pedigree (D) incorrectly specifies that the affected stillborn cousin is related through his mother.

28–29. The answers are: 28-C, 29-B. *(Gelehrter, pp 27–29. Thompson, 5/e, pp 53–57.)* Twins are indicated by connection to the marriage bar by *diagonal lines* with monozygous (identical) twins being connected together. The dizygous twins represented in figure C that accompanies the question are discordant since one is affected with a disorder and the other is not. This might be expected, since dizygous twins are like siblings—that is, first-degree relatives share 50 percent of their genes. Monozygous twins are usually concordant for Mendelian or chromosomal diseases but may be discordant for multifactorial diseases. If one twin is affected with a multifactorial birth defect, such as cleft palate, there is only a 40 percent chance that the other twin with identical genes will be affected. This indicates the importance of environmental factors, including the intrauterine environment, in multifactorial diseases. The divorce (*slash of marriage bar*) and adopted out (*outward bracket*) symbols are shown in B of the figure, and spontaneous abortion (*small filled circle*) is indicated in E.

30–31. The answers are: 30-B, 31-D. *(Gelehrter, pp 27–30. Thompson, 5/e, p 2.)* Chromosomal disorders, because they often produce severe phenotypes, have a larger incidence at birth (0.5 to 0.7 percent in newborn surveys) than in older age-groups. As infectious diseases have been conquered, chronic diseases have become an important factor in pediatric hospital admissions; genetic diseases account for 10 to 25 percent of cases in three surveys. Most are multifactorial disorders that include common birth defects and diseases with a genetic predisposition, such as schizophrenia, alcoholism, or diabetes mellitus. Mendelian disorders may produce subtle phenotypes in the newborn but have major consequences in later life (e.g., Marfan syndrome and familial hypercholesterolemia). Current incidence figures are underestimates that will increase once widespread genetic screening is available for complex diseases.

32–36. The answers are: 32-E, 33-J, 34-A, 35-G, 36-D. *(Gelehrter, pp 27–29. Thompson, 5/e, pp 53–57.)* The numbering of generations (*Roman numerals*) and individuals (*Arabic numerals*) allows easy reference to individual data. Often it is more legible and convenient to draw and number the pedigree, then to tabulate individual traits in a key as shown in the figure

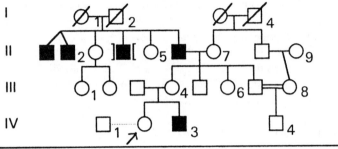

Bateson family
IV-2 Diane Bateson, age 23   III-7 John Fisher, age 43
III-4 Paula Bateson, age 48   - - - - - - -
II-6 Ronald Fisher, age 71   - - - - - - -

above. Only Diane's family is represented because it is relevant to the medical question. The pedigree suggests X-linked recessive inheritance.

37– 46. The answers are: 37-C, 38-M, 39-0, 40-R, 41-Q, 42-D, 43-I, 44-H, 45-G, 46-N. *(Gelehrter, pp 27–29. Thompson, 5/e, pp 53–57.)* A pedigree is a scientific genealogy in which individuals and relationships are symbolized precisely. The proband (or propositus), who is identified by an *arrow,* is the person first ascertained with the disease of interest or the person who requests information; he or she is also termed a *consultand.* Males are represented by *squares* and females by *circles;* numbers inside the symbol provide a short-hand method to indicate several individuals at once. A *diamond* may be used when the sex is unknown. *Filled-in symbols* represent affected individuals. Carriers of X-linked disorders (females) are indicated by a *dotted circle;* carriers of autosomal recessive diseases may be indicated by a *half-filled symbol.* *Brackets* are used to represent adoption; the direction of the brackets show whether the individual was adopted in or out.

Individual symbols in a pedigree are connected in ways that indicate family relationships. Each row of symbols represents a generation, and a union is indicated by a *dotted line* (no marriage), a *solid line* (marriage), *solid line with a hatch* (divorce), or a *double line* (consanguineous marriage, e.g., parents are first cousins). Offspring are drawn in the order of birth with prenatal deaths indicated by *small symbols.* Twins are connected to the marriage bar by *diagonal lines* and connected to each other if they are identical. For clarity, generations (Roman numerals) and individuals (Arabic numerals) may be numbered.

Chromosomal Inheritance

DIRECTIONS: Each question below contains four or five suggested responses. Select the **one best** response to each question.

47. Chromosomal imbalance is most frequent during which of the following stages of human development?

(A) Embryonic
(B) Fetal
(C) Neonatal
(D) Childhood
(E) Adult

48. During mitosis, the parent and daughter cells have which of the following chromosome compositions?

(A) Haploid
(B) Diploid
(C) Parent cell—diploid; daughter cell—haploid
(D) Triploid
(E) Tetraploid

49. The standard karyotype is performed by photomicroscopy of cells at which mitotic stage?

(A) Interphase
(B) Prophase
(C) Metaphase
(D) Anaphase
(E) Telophase

50. A couple is referred to the physician because the first three pregnancies have ended in spontaneous abortion. Chromosomal analysis reveals that the wife has two cell lines in her blood, one with a missing X chromosome (45,X) and the other normal (46,XX). Her chromosomal constitution can be described as

(A) chimeric
(B) monoploid
(C) trisomic
(D) mosaic
(E) euploid

51. A child with cleft palate, a heart defect, and extra fifth fingers is found to have 46 chromosomes with extra material on one homologue of the chromosome 5 pair. This chromosomal abnormality is best described by which of the following terms?

(A) Polyploidy
(B) Rearrangement
(C) Aneuploidy
(D) Mosaicism
(E) Sex chromosome aneuploidy

52. The cell labeled A in the figure below is best described by which of the following terms?

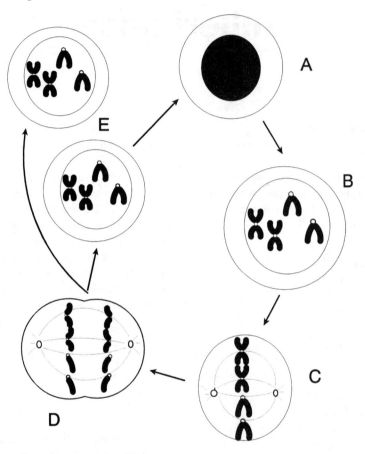

(A) Meiotic I interphase, haploid
(B) Mitotic telophase, diploid
(C) Meiotic I metaphase, diploid
(D) Mitotic interphase, diploid
(E) Mitotic anaphase, diploid

53. Standard karyotyping involves which of the following sequences of methods?

(A) Frozen blood sample, leukocyte culture for 12–48 hours, metaphase arrest with lectins, hypotonic saline treatment, slide spreading, staining to produce bands, and photomicroscopy

(B) Anticoagulated blood sample, stimulation of cell division with lectins, immediate metaphase arrest with colchicine, hypotonic saline treatment, slide spreading, staining to produce bands, and photomicroscopy

(C) Clotted blood sample, leukocyte culture for 12–48 hours, metaphase arrest with lectins, hypotonic saline treatment, slide spreading, staining to produce bands, and photomicroscopy

(D) Frozen blood sample, immediate metaphase arrest with colchicine, hypotonic saline treatment, slide spreading, staining to produce bands, and photomicroscopy

(E) Anticoagulated blood sample, lectin stimulation, leukocyte culture for 12–48 hours, metaphase arrest with colchicine, hypotonic saline treatment, slide spreading, staining to produce bands, and photomicroscopy

54. The paired homologues in a normal karyotype can be represented as (4a4b), (15a15b), (21a21b), and so on. Which of the following notations accurately reflects the sorting of two chromosome pairs during normal female meiosis?

(A) Primary oocytes (4a4a, 15b15b); secondary oocytes (4a, 15b); ova same as secondary oocytes

(B) Primary oocytes (4a4b, 15a15b); secondary oocytes (4a4b, 15a15b); ova (4a, 15b), (4a, 15a), (4b, 15a), or (4b, 15b)

(C) Primary oocytes (4a, 4b, 15a15b); secondary oocytes (4a4b) or (15a15b); ova same as secondary oocytes

(D) Primary oocytes (4a4b, 15a15b); secondary oocytes (4a4b, 15a15b); ova same as secondary oocytes

(E) Primary oocytes (4a4b, 15a15b); secondary oocytes (4a, 15b), (4a, 15a), (4b, 15a), or (4b, 15b); ova same as secondary oocytes

20 Genetics

55. The Prader-Willi and Angelman syndromes can arise from identical deletions on the proximal long arm of chromosome 15. In Prader-Willi syndrome, the deletion is always on the paternal chromosome 15, while in Angelman syndrome, it is always on the maternal chromosome 15. For small deletions, polymerase chain reaction (PCR) amplification of variably sized (polymorphic) DNA fragments within the deletion may be necessary to determine which parental chromosome is affected. The lettered diagrams below represent gels that separate amplified chromosome 15 DNA fragments by size from a mother (M), father (F), and child (C). Which diagram is diagnostic of Prader-Willi syndrome in the child?

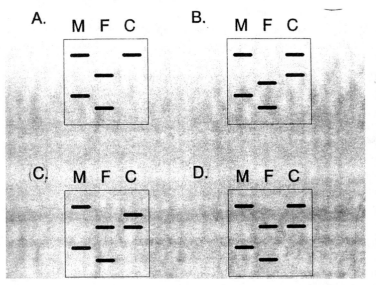

56. The paired homologues in a normal karyotype can be represented as (4a4b), (15a15b), (21a21b), and so on. Which of the following notations represents the possibilities for an abnormal gamete caused by nondisjunction at meiotic division II?

(A) (21a21a) or (21b21b)
(B) (21a21b) or (21a21a)
(C) (21a21b) or (21b21b)
(D) (21b)
(E) (21a21b)

57. A 10-year-old boy is referred to the physician because of a learning disability and lack of motivation in school. Physical examination is normal except for single palmar creases (a minor anomaly) and curved fifth fingers (clinodactyly). Chromosomal analysis reveals a 47,XYY karyotype. The error in meiosis that produces this karyotype is best described by

(A) meiosis division I of paternal spermatogenesis
(B) meiosis division I of maternal oogenesis
(C) meiosis division II of paternal spermatogenesis
(D) meiosis division II of maternal oogenesis
(E) meiosis division II in either parent

58. Fluorescent in situ hybridization (FISH) analysis is a technique in which DNA probes are used to visualize loci on chromosomes. Interphase chromosomes prior to DNA replication yield one hybridization signal per chromosome with single-copy FISH probes (i.e., probes for genes that occur once per genome). Assuming that a separate FISH signal is generated for each DNA strand present in a chromosome, expected FISH results after hybridization to a section of the testis include which of the following? (PSI = primary spermatocytes [interphase]; PSP = primary spermatocytes [prophase]; SSI = secondary spermatocytes [interphase]; and SSP = secondary spermatocytes [prophase])

(A) PSI-2 signals, PSP-4, SSI-2, SSP-4, sperm-1
(B) PSI-2 signals, PSP-4, SSI-2, SSP-2, sperm-1
(C) PSI-2 signals, PSP-4, SSI-2, SSP-2, sperm-1
(D) PSI-4 signals, PSP-4, SSI-2, SSP-2, sperm-1
(E) PSI-2 signals, PSP-4, SSI-4, SSP-2, sperm-1

59. Division of the centromeres involves which of the following stages?

(A) Mitotic prophase, meiotic I metaphase
(B) Mitotic telophase, meiotic I metaphase
(C) Mitotic metaphase, meiotic I metaphase
(D) Mitotic metaphase, meiotic II metaphase
(E) Mitotic prophase, meiotic II metaphase

60. Which of the following karyotypes is an example of aneuploidy?

(A) 46,XX
(B) 23,X
(C) 69,XXX
(D) 92,XXXX
(E) 90,XX

61. The cytogenetic term "6q+" refers to

(A) 46,XX,dup(6q)
(B) extra chromosome material derived from the long arm of chromosome 6
(C) 46,XX,dup(6p)
(D) extra chromosome material, origin unspecified, attached to the long arm of chromosome 6
(E) 47,XX,+6

62. The proper cytogenetic notation for a female with Down syndrome mosaicism is

(A) 46,XX,+21/46,XY
(B) 47,XY,+21
(C) 47,XXX/46,XX
(D) 47,XX,+21/46,XX
(E) 47,XX,+21(46,XX)

DIRECTIONS: Each numbered question or incomplete statement below is NEGATIVELY phrased. Select the **one best** lettered response.

63. The Prader-Willi syndrome involves a voracious appetite, obesity, short stature, hypogonadism, and mental disability. At least 50 percent of Prader-Willi patients have a small deletion on the proximal long arm of chromosome 15. In detecting the Prader-Willi deletion, all the following techniques would be helpful EXCEPT

(A) prometaphase analysis of peripheral blood from the patient
(B) Southern blotting of patient DNA, using single-copy DNA segments isolated from the deleted region as probes
(C) polymerase chain reaction (PCR), using primers that amplify single-copy DNA segments from the deleted region
(D) rapid karyotyping of bone marrow from the patient
(E) fluorescent in situ hybridization (FISH) analysis of peripheral blood lymphocytes, using fluorescent DNA probes from the deleted region

64. Loss of heterozygosity in tumors is caused by all the following EXCEPT

(A) nondisjunction producing monosomy
(B) uniparental disomy
(C) interstitial deletion
(D) translocation
(E) polyploidy

65. Clinical indications for karyotyping include all the following EXCEPT

(A) multiple malformations in a newborn
(B) single malformation in a newborn
(C) mental retardation of unknown etiology
(D) offspring with a chromosomal rearrangement
(E) recurrent pregnancy loss

DIRECTIONS: Each group of questions below consists of lettered headings followed by a set of numbered items. For each numbered item select the **one** lettered heading with which it is **most** closely associated. Each lettered heading may be used **once, more than once or not at all.**

Questions 66–68

Match each clinical situation below with the appropriate risk figure.

(A) 1/10,000
(B) 1/600
(C) 1/100
(D) 1/10
(E) 1

66. The risk for a newborn to have Down syndrome

67. The theoretical risk for a 21/21 translocation carrier to have a child with Down syndrome

68. The risk for parents of a trisomy 21 child to have a second offspring with a chromosomal abnormality

Questions 69–71

Match each individual below with the correct karyotype.

(A) 46,XY
(B) 23,X
(C) 69,XXY
(D) 47,XX+21
(E) 92,XXXX

69. Haploid individual

70. Diploid individual

71. Triploid individual

Questions 72–74

For each of the genetic results described below, select the appropriate physical (chromosomal) basis.

(A) Homologous recombination
(B) Heterochromatin
(C) Separation of chromosomal homologues (reduction division)
(D) Meiotic or mitotic nondisjunction
(E) Mitotic nondisjunction

72. Mendel's law of independent assortment

73. Germinal mosaicism

74. Somatic mosaicism

Questions 75–77

Match each of the genetic conditions below with the correct cytogenetic notation.

(A) 47,XX,+21
(B) 45,X
(C) 47,XXX
(D) 47,XY,+21
(E) 45,XX−21

75. Male with trisomy 21 (Down syndrome)

76. Female with monosomy X (Turner syndrome)

77. Female with monosomy 21

Questions 78–80

Match each cytogenetic description with the appropriate lettered diagram.

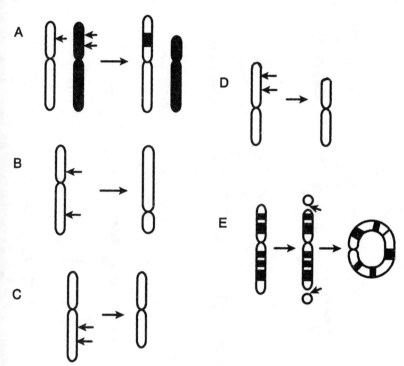

78. Insertional translocation (nonreciprocal)

79. Pericentric inversion

80. Interstitial deletion of long arm

Questions 81–83

Match each cytogenetic notation with the appropriate lettered diagram in the previous question group.

81. 46,XX,r(7)(p25q23)

82 46,XX,del(6)(q15q25)

83. 46,XX,inv(7)(p14q25)

Questions 84–86

Match each cytogenetic description with the appropriate lettered diagram.

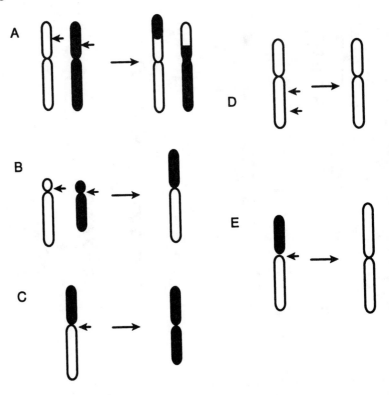

84. Isochromosome (short arm)

85. Robertsonian translocation

86. Reciprocal translocation

Questions 87–89

Match each cytogenetic notation with the correct lettered diagram in the previous question group.

87. 46,XX,i(6q)

88. 45,XX,t(14q15q)

89. 46,XY,t(7p22;9p15)

Questions 90–91

For each of the mechanisms listed below, select the disorder that is most likely to result.

(A) 45,X/46,XX
(B) 45,X
(C) 47,XXX
(D) 47,XYY
(E) 47,XXY

90. Nondisjunction at meiosis II only

91. Nondisjunction after fertilization

Questions 92–93

Match each cytogenetic notation with the correct phenotype.

(A) Patient with Down syndrome
(B) Translocation carrier with risk for a child with Down syndrome
(C) Patient with Patau syndrome
(D) Translocation carrier with risk for a child with Patau syndrome
(E) Patient with Down syndrome mosaicism

92. 45,XX,t(21q21q)

93. 46,XX,t(21q21q)

Questions 94–96

Match each cytogenetic notation below with the appropriate description.

(A) One Barr body
(B) No Barr bodies
(C) Two inactive X chromosomes
(D) Three inactive X chromosomes
(E) Four inactive X chromosomes

94. 46,XY

95. 46,XX

96. 49,XXXXX

Questions 97–98

Match each cytogenetic notation with the correct lettered mechanism of rearrangement and segregation.

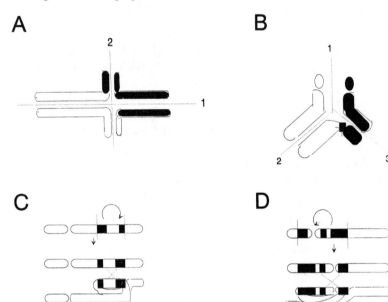

97. 46,XX,t(13q14q)

98. 46,XX,inv dup(6)(q33q23)

Questions 99–100

Match each cytogenetic notation below with the correct karyotype.

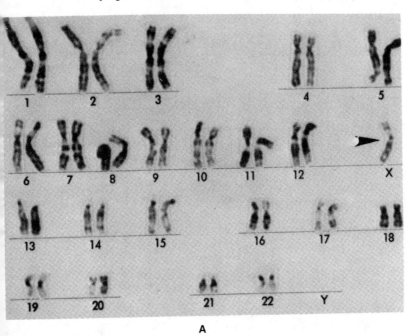

A

99. 47,XX+21

100. 46,XY,t(14q21q)

(Illustrations continue next page)

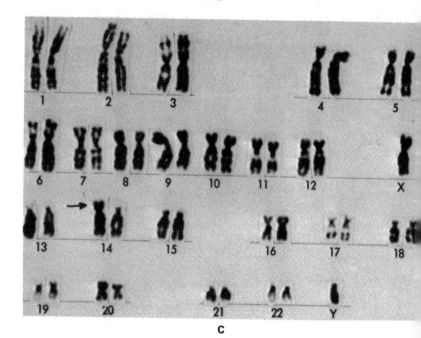

B

C

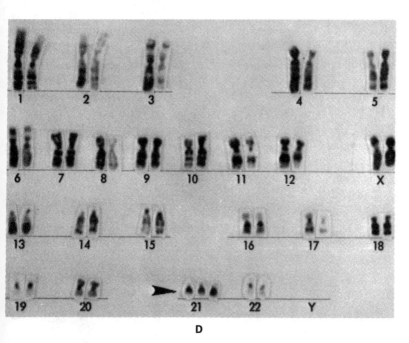

D

Questions 101–102

Match each clinical diagnosis with the appropriate karyotype in the previous question group.

101. Translocation Down syndrome

102. Triploidy

Questions 103–107

Match each term listed below with the chromosomal structure that best explains it.

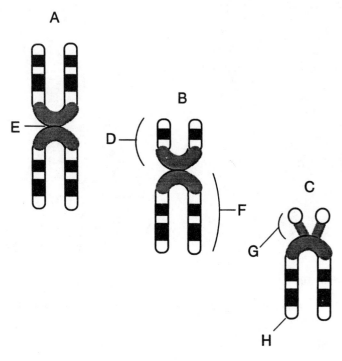

103. Submetacentric chromosome

104. Short arm, or p

105. Centromere

106. Long arm, or q

107. Chromosome band (light)

Questions 108–112

   Match each cytogenetic notation below with the correct karyotype.

108. 46,XY,del(4p)

109. 18q−

110. 5p−

111. 3q+

112. 46,XY,14p+

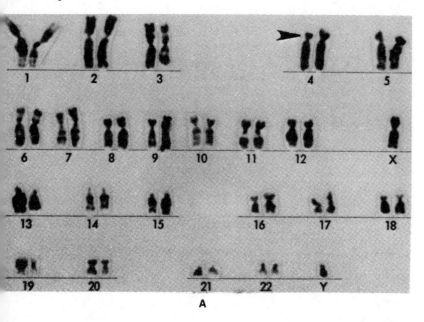

A

(Illustrations continue next page)

B

C

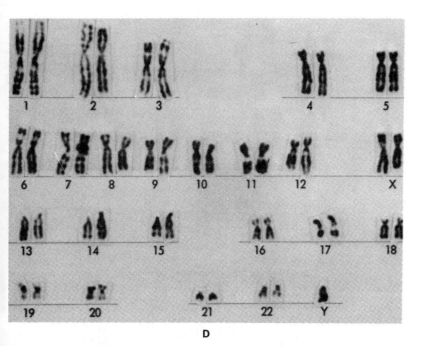

D

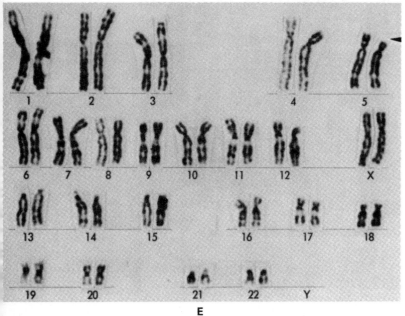

E

(Illustrations continue next page)

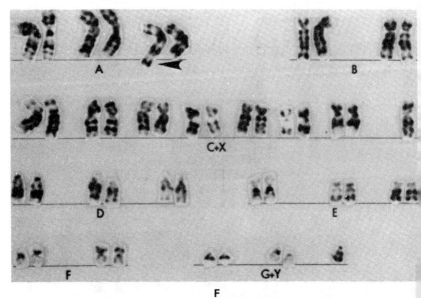

F

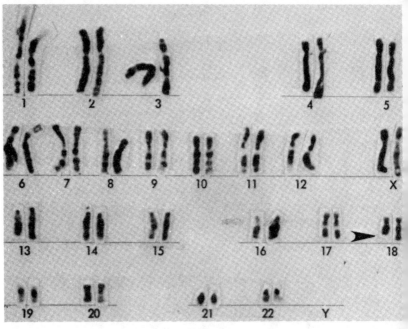

G

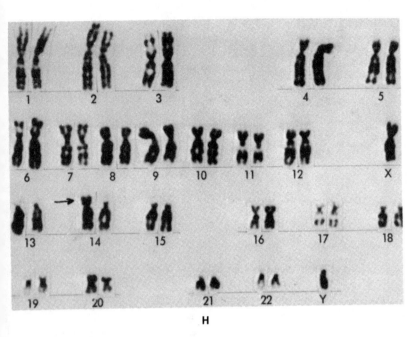

H

Questions 113–117

Match each clinical syndrome below with the correct karyotype in the previous question group.

113. Cri du chat syndrome

114. Dup(3q) syndrome

115. Klinefelter syndrome

116. 47,XYY syndrome

117. Translocation Down syndrome

Questions 118–122

Match each description below with the correct stage of meiosis depicted in the figure.

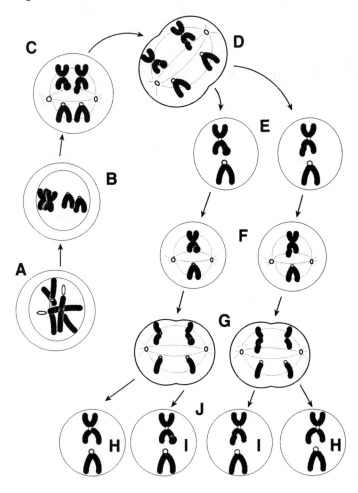

118. Tetrads

119. Synapsis

120. Segregation of homologues

121. Meiosis division II metaphase

122. Separation of sister chromatids

Questions 123–127

Match each of the cell types below with the correct stage of meiosis depicted in the figure in the previous question group.

123. Primary spermatocytes

124. Secondary oocytes

125. Egg at ovulation

126. Mature ovum

127. Haploid gametes

Chromosomal Inheritance

Answers

47. The answer is A. *(Gelehrter, pp 159–192. Thompson, 5/e, pp 201–230.)* Chromosomal aberrations occur in approximately 1 in 200 live-born infants, 4 percent of stillbirths, and 50 percent of all first-trimester abortuses. At least 15 to 20 percent of conceptions result in spontaneous abortion (miscarriage) during the first trimester (i.e., < 12 weeks' gestation). Although the exact frequency of chromosomal anomalies in human embryos (i.e., < 8 weeks' gestation) is unknown, the numbers above indicate a substantial frequency of at least 7.5 percent.

48. The answer is B. *(Gelehrter, p 20. Thompson, 5/e, pp 13–30.)* The number of different chromosomes that occur in an organism is called the chromosome number and is represented by *n*. Ploidy refers to multiples of the chromosome number that occur in a cell: n = monoploid or haploid, $2n$ = diploid, $3n$ = triploid, and $4n$ = tetraploid. Mitosis is a mechanism by which the paired, diploid chromosomes of a parental cell are duplicated to form two diploid daughter cells. Unlike the first cell division in meiosis, there is no change in chromosome number.

49. The answer is C. *(Gelehrter, pp 159–162. Thompson, 5/e, pp 13–30.)* The standard karyotype is an arrangement of chromosomes from one cell that is undergoing division at metaphase. At other mitotic stages, the chromosomes are not sufficiently condensed or are too dispersed to allow counting and comparison of pairs under the microscope. After growth, metaphase arrest, separation, hypotonic treatment, and fixing of white blood cells, smearing on a slide yields only about 3 percent of cells that can be analyzed (metaphase spreads). In high resolution chromosome analysis, less condensed chromosomes in late prophase may be analyzed (prometaphase analysis); however, this process is extremely time-consuming and usually requires focus on a particular chromosome region (e.g., chromosome 15 in a patient suspected of Prader-Willi syndrome, a condition marked by obesity and mental retardation).

50. The answer is D. *(Gelehrter, pp 159–189. Thompson, 5/e, p 217.)* The case described in the question represents one of the commoner chromosomal causes of reproductive failure, Turner mosaicism. Turner syndrome represents a pattern of anomalies, including short stature, heart defects, and infertility. Turner syndrome is often associated with a 45,X karyotype (monosomy X) in females, but mosaicism (i.e., two or more cell lines in the same individual with different karyotypes) is common. However, chimerism (i.e., two cell lines in an individual arising from different zygotes, such as fraternal twins who do not separate) is extremely rare. Trisomy refers to three copies of one chromosome; euploidy, to a normal chromosome number; and monoploidy, to one set of chromosomes (haploidy in humans).

51. The answer is B. *(Gelehrter, pp 159–189. Thompson, 5/e, pp 201–214.)* Chromosomal abnormalities may involve changes in number (i.e., polyploidy and aneuploidy) or changes in structure (i.e., rearrangements, such as translocations, rings, and inversions). Extra material (i.e., extra chromatin) seen on chromosome 5 implies recombination of chromosome 5 DNA with that of another chromosome to produce a rearranged chromosome. Since this rearranged chromosome 5 takes the place of a normal chromosome 5, there is no change in number of the autosomes (nonsex chromosomes) or sex chromosomes (X and Y chromosomes). The question implies that all cells karyotyped from the patient (usually 11–25 cells) had the same chromosomal constitution, ruling out mosaicism. The patient's clinical findings are similar to those occurring in trisomy 13, suggesting that the extra material on chromosome 5 is derived from chromosome 13, producing an unbalanced karyotype called dup(13) or partial trisomy 13.

52. The answer is D. *(Gelehrter, pp 20–21. Thompson, 5/e, pp 13–30.)* The figure that accompanies the question depicts mitosis with its stages of interphase (A), prophase (B), metaphase (C), telophase (D), and division to yield daughter cells (E). Mitosis is the mechanism by which somatic cells duplicate each pair of chromosomes to produce identical copies in diploid daughter cells. At mitotic interphase, the diploid chromatin is dispersed and actively transcribed prior to DNA replication and condensation. Meiosis involves two successive divisions to produce haploid gametes.

53. The answer is E. *(Gelehrter, pp 159–162. Thompson, 5/e, pp 13–30.)* Standard karyotyping is performed on the most accessible tissue, which in children and adults is peripheral blood. Because nucleated cells must be used, anticoagulated blood is required so that leukocytes can be separated from red blood cells by centrifugation. To obtain metaphase spreads, dividing cells are obtained by lectin (usually phytohemagglutinin) stimulation, leukocyte culture for 12–48 hours, and metaphase arrest with colchicine. Hypotonic treatment is necessary to rupture cells and nuclei when they are smeared on slides; various staining methods then highlight the chromosomes for microscopy. Clotted or frozen blood cannot be used. Rapid karyotyping requires cells that are already dividing, such as bone marrow, or for infants, umbilical cord blood.

54. The answer is E. *(Gelehrter, pp 19–23. Thompson, 5/e, pp 13–30.)* The first meiotic division is called a *reduction division* because the 46 paired chromosomes replicate then separate by homologues into daughter cells with 23 chromosomes (still diploid DNA content). Individual chromosome pairs (i.e., 4a4b and 15a15b) line up randomly at the first meiotic metaphase. Consequently, daughter cells can have any one of four possible combinations: (4a, 15a), (4a, 15b), (4b, 15a), or (4b, 15b). After the reduction division (meiosis I), secondary spermatocytes or oocytes divide without DNA replication (meiosis II) to produce haploid gametes: (4a, 15a), (4a, 15b), (4b, 15a), or (4b, 15b). The random sorting of 23 chromosome homologues allows for more than 8 million combinations in gametes and can be amplified even more by recombination between homologues at meiosis I metaphase (*synapsis*).

55. The answer is A. *(Thompson, 5/e, pp 92–95.)* Diagram A in the figure that accompanies the question shows only one band in lane C, indicating that a DNA fragment of one size has been amplified by the polymerase chain reaction (PCR). This fragment is the same size as one of the maternal DNA fragments, indicating that the child has inherited this fragment (allele) from its mother. Neither of the father's fragments are present, suggesting that the paternal chromosome 15 has been deleted in the child. An alternative explanation would be inheritance of two copies of the same maternal 15 chromosome (uniparental disomy); however, in that case, the child's band should be of double density. Nonpaternity is suggested by diagram B, where the child has a fragment that does not match up with the father's. Diagram C suggests nonmaternity (i.e., switching in the nursery); the paternal match may represent a common fragment size in the population. Diagram D illustrates normal biparental inheritance of the DNA fragment alleles.

56. The answer is A. *(Gelehrter, pp 19–23. Thompson, 5/e, pp 13–30.)* The chromosomal homologues are separated in the first meiotic division (meiosis I), producing secondary oocytes or spermatocytes with one maternally derived or one paternally derived homologue (sister chromatids attached by a centromere). The paired chromosomes of each primary germ cell (21a21b) segregate into two secondary germ cells (21a or 21b) and form four gametes (21a or 21b) during meiosis. Nondisjunction at meiosis I produces secondary germ cells with both homologues (21a21b), while nondisjunction at meiosis II produces disomic gametes (24,X or 24,Y) with two copies of the same homologue (21a21a or 21b21b). Gametes with a single homologue (21a or 21b) are normal (23,X or 23,Y). Fertilization of a disomic 21 gamete by a normal gamete produces trisomy 21.

57. The answer is C. *(Gelehrter, pp 19–23. Thompson, 5/e, pp 13–30.)* The sex chromosomes with differently named homologues allow easy visualization of chromosome sorting during meiosis. Female meiosis only involves X chromosomes; thus, Y chromosomal abnormalities must arise during paternal meiosis or occur spontaneously in offspring. Nondisjunction at paternal meiosis I produces XY secondary spermatocytes and a 24,XY gamete. Fertilization with a 23,X ovum yields a 47,XXY individual (Klinefelter syndrome). Only nondisjunction at paternal meiosis II produces a 24,YY gamete that yields a 47,XYY individual after fertilization. As in the patient described in the question, 47,XYY individuals often have minimal physical or intellectual disabilities.

58. The answer is B. *(Gelehrter, pp 19–23. Thompson, 5/e, pp 13–30.)* Interphase diploid cells, including primordial germ cells, yield two hybridization signals for a fluorescent in situ hybridization (FISH) probe that recognizes one locus per chromosome. DNA replication occurs during the S phase of cell division, so that by prophase (beginning of chromosomal condensation), there will be two DNA strands per chromosome (sister chromatids). FISH probes yield four hybridization signals for the replicated chromosomes in prophase of mitosis or meiosis I. During meiosis I, the primary spermatocytes undergo division with segregation of one replicated homologue into each daughter cell. These secondary spermatocytes yield two hybridization signals (one homologue, two sister chromatids). Since there is no DNA replication in meiosis II, two signals are also obtained for secondary spermatocytes in prophase. During meiosis II division, centromeres divide to segregate one sister chromatid into each gamete. Single-copy FISH probes yield one signal per normal sperm cell.

59. The answer is D. *(Gelehrter, pp 19–23. Thompson, 5/e, pp 13–30.)* Division of centromeres occurs when sister chromatids are separated into daughter cells. This does not occur during meiotic division I, where the two homologues (sister chromatids plus centromere) line up on the metaphase plate (synapsis). Division at this time separates homologues rather than sister chromatids. Centromeric division occurs during mitotic metaphase and meiotic II metaphase, partitioning sister chromatids and producing identical chromosomal complements in daughter cells.

60. The answer is E. *(Gelehrter, pp 159–192. Thompson, 5/e, pp 201–230.)* Aneuploidy involves extra or missing chromosomes that do not arise as increments of the haploid chromosome number *n*. Polyploidy involves multiples of *n*, such as triploidy (3*n* = 69,XXX) or tetraploidy (4*n* = 92,XXXX). Diploidy (46,XX) and haploidy (23,X) are normal karyotypes in gametes and somatic cells, respectively. A 90,XX karyotype represents tetraploidy with two missing X chromosomes, which has been seen in one patient who had features that resembled those of Turner syndrome.

61. The answer is D. *(Gelehrter, pp 159–192. Thompson, 5/e, pp 201–230.)* The term "6q+" is shorthand for a karyotype showing extra chromosomal material on the long arm of chromosome 6. The origin of the extra material is not specified; therefore, clinical correlation or additional banding and molecular studies are needed to define from which chromosome the extra material is derived. When rearrangements are found, it is necessary to obtain karyotypes from the parents. This may define the extra material if the parent carries a reciprocal translocation (i.e., one of the parental chromosomes is deleted for the material that is attached to 6q). The notation dup(6q) specifies that the extra material is derived from the long arm of chromosome 6. The notation 47,XX+6 implies trisomy for the entire number 6 chromosome.

62. The answer is D. *(Gelehrter, pp 159–192. Thompson, 5/e, pp 201–230.)* Mosaicism occurs when a chromosomal anomaly affects one of several precursor cells of an embryo or tissue. The two or more karyotypes that characterize the mosaic cells are separated by a slash in cytogenetic notation. The notation 47,XX,+21 denotes a cell line typical of a female with trisomy 21 (Down syndrome), while 46,XX is the karyotype expected for a normal female.

63. The answer is D. *(Gelehrter, pp 159–192. Thompson, 5/e, pp 201–230.)* The Prader-Willi deletion is quite small and is not usually detected by standard metaphase karyotyping. Standard karyotypes typically display about 300 bands over the 23 chromosomes or about 10 bands on chromosome 10. Prometaphase karyotyping evaluates less condensed chromosomes in early metaphase, revealing 500 to 1000 bands over the entire karyotype. Prometaphase banding detects most Prader-Willi deletions (*microdeletions*); however, some deletions require even more sensitive techniques that test for the absence of DNA segments within the deleted region (*submicroscopic deletions*).

DNA analysis can be performed laboriously via Southern blotting, less laboriously by polymerase chain reaction (PCR) analysis, and most efficiently by fluorescent in situ hybridization (FISH) analysis on the same leukocytes used for karyotyping. Rapid karyotyping of bone marrow samples usually gives poor resolution that is adequate for detecting aneuploidy but inadequate for subtle deletions seen in patients with the Prader-Willi syndrome.

64. The answer is E. *(Gelehrter, pp 229–254. Thompson, 5/e, pp 365–382.)* The Knudson hypothesis suggested a two-hit model for cancers that show genetic predisposition. The two hits comprise a first mutation present in germ cells and a second mutation acquired in somatic cells of the susceptible tissue. If the two hits affect one genetic locus, then the germ cell is heterozygous (i.e., one abnormal allele) and the somatic cell becomes homozygous (i.e., two abnormal alleles, which denotes a loss of heterozygosity). Physical evidence for this second hit includes chromosomal mechanisms that remove one chromosome and, thus, the remaining normal (suppressor) allele. Evidence of these mechanisms can include complete loss of the chromosome (monosomy); deletion of the suppressor gene region (interstitial or internal deletion); abnormal cell division that yields two copies of the same chromosome homologue in a daughter cell (uniparental disomy); and a translocation that disrupts the suppressor gene. Polyploidy involves multiplication of the haploid number *n*. This is a mechanism that produces more normal suppressor alleles rather than deleting one.

65. The answer is B. *(Gelehrter, p 187.)* The hallmarks of chromosomal disease in children are multiple malformations and mental retardation. Frequently growth is impaired, and the facial appearance is unusual. Parents of children with chromosomal rearrangements (i.e., translocations, deletions, or duplications) must be karyotyped to determine if they are carriers of balanced translocations. Approximately 5 percent of couples with more than three first-trimester abortions have balanced chromosomal rearrangements as a cause for pregnancy loss or infertility. Chromosomal analysis should also be considered in patients with unexplained mental retardation, particularly if they have an unusual appearance or a family history of mental retardation. The child with a single birth defect (e.g., cleft palate or dislocated hip) rarely has a chromosomal abnormality unless there are undetected minor or internal anomalies that comprise a malformation syndrome.

66–68. The answers are: 66-B, 67-E, 68-C. *(Gelehrter, pp 159–192. Thompson, 5/e, pp 201–230.)* The incidence of Down syndrome at birth is approximately 1 in 600 live-born children with 95 percent being trisomy 21.

About 4 percent of Down syndrome patients have translocations that mandate parental karyotyping to determine if one of the parents is a balanced translocation carrier. The remaining 1 percent are mosaics, meaning that certain tissues are mixtures of trisomy 21 and normal cells. Translocation carriers have a 5 to 20 percent risk for unbalanced offspring with female carriers in general at higher risk than male carriers. Offspring of translocation 21/21 carriers should in theory all have Down syndrome, although some carriers have had normal children. The empiric risk for parents with a trisomy 21 child is 1/100 for a second child with chromosomal aneuploidy.

69–71. The answers are: 69-B, 70-A, 71-C. *(Gelehrter, pp 159–192. Thompson, 5/e, pp 201–230.)* There are 23 different chromosomes in normal human gametes comprised of 22 autosomes and 1 X or Y sex chromosome. Cytogenetic notation indicates the total number of chromosomes, followed by the sex chromosomal constitution. At fertilization, 23,X or 23,Y gametes (i.e., haploid cells) unite to form a diploid zygote (46,XX or 46,XY, i.e., euloidy). Errors in meiosis may produce gametes with one missing or extra chromosome, which after fertilization generates an embryo with 45 or 47 chromosomes (e.g., 47,XX+21), which is called aneuploidy. Many aneuploid embryos abort in the first trimester, but trisomies 13, 18, and 21 and monosomy X may survive and present as neonates. Rarely, gametes contain an additional chromosome complement such that they have $2n$ or $3n$ chromosomes where $n = 23$. The resulting embryo has $3n$ (69,XXY) or $4n$ (92,XXXX) chromosomes, producing a triploid or tetraploid fetus with severe birth defects.

72–74. The answers are: 72-C, 73-D, 74-E. *(Gelehrter, pp 159–192. Thompson, 5/e, pp 201–230.)* Mendel's laws of segregation and independent assortment received direct physical verification when technology allowed visualization of chromosomal segregation during meiosis. Failure of segregation (*nondisjunction*) at meiosis I or II generates abnormal gametes; if this happens only in selected germ cells, the gonad will contain a mixture of karyotypically normal and abnormal gametes (*germinal mosaicism*). Such individuals may have several children with genetic diseases that normally have a very low recurrence risk (e.g., trisomy 21). If nondisjunction occurs during mitosis, then the embryonic or adult tissue will be a composite of karyotypically normal and abnormal cells (*somatic mosaicism*). Homologous recombination between chromosomal homologues generates new combinations of alleles but not chromosomal rearrangements. Nonhomologous recombination can create chromosomal translocations and inversions. Heterochromatin refers to densely staining chromosomal regions composed of highly repetitive or satellite DNA.

75–77. The answers are: 75-D, 76-B, 77-E. *(Gelehrter, pp 159–192. Thompson, 5/e, pp 201–230.)* Cytogenetic notation provides the chromosome number (e.g., 46), the sex chromosomes, and a shorthand description of anomalies. Examples include the following: 47,XX+21 indicates a female with trisomy 21; 45,X indicates a female with monosomy X; or 45,XX−21 indicates a female with monosomy 21. Note the absence of spaces between symbols, and the use of 45,X or 47,XXX for sex chromosomal aneuploidy rather than the more awkward 45,XX−X or 47,XX+X.

78–80. The answers are: 78-A, 79-B, 80-C. *(Gelehrter, pp 159–192. Thompson, 5/e, pp 201–230.)* Ring chromosomes (diagram E), interstitial deletions (diagrams C [long arm] and D [short arm]), and pericentric inversions (diagram B) are examples of intrachromosomal rearrangements in which breaks or crossovers unite different regions of the same chromosome. The inverted segment contains the centromere in *pericentric* inversions but not in *paracentric* inversions. Translocations (diagram A) are rearrangements that join regions of different chromosomes together. They are *reciprocal* when there is exchange between two chromosomes and *nonreciprocal* when there is a one-way transfer of a chromosome fragment. Donor chromosomes may lose material from internal regions (interstitial deletions) or from ends (terminal deletions), just as recipient chromosomes may have insertional or terminal duplications.

81–83. The answers are: 81-E, 82-C, 83-B. *(Gelehrter, pp 163–171. Thompson, 5/e, pp 201–214.)* The abbreviations *inv, dup, del,* and *r* describe inverted, duplicated, deleted, and ring chromosome segments, respectively. The segment involved is delimited by the bands at its borders. Bands are numbered according to their distance from the centromere: band 3p3 is distal (nearer the telomere) and band 3p1 is proximal (nearer the centromere) on the short arm of chromosome 3. Better techniques reveal sub-bands within larger bands that are numbered similarly (e.g., 3p11, 3p12). The cytogenetic notation r(7)(p25q23) describes breakpoints in chromosome 7 at bands p25 (short arm) and q23 (long arm) with subsequent joining to form a ring (diagram E). Breakpoints in the long arm indicate a long-arm deletion (diagram C), and breakpoints in both arms indicate a pericentric inversion (diagram B). The insertional translocation in diagram A requires a more detailed notation, such as 46,XX,−7,−9,+der(7)(7pter—>7p13::9p13—>p25::7p13—>7qter),+del(9) (p13p25). The notation indicates replacement of normal chromosomes (−7, −9), with a derived (der) 7 and deleted (del) 9 chromosome. The exact rearrangement is then described from the short-arm terminus (pter) to the long-arm terminus (qter). Breakpoints are indicated by *colons* (::), while *arrows* indicate preserved chromosome regions.

48 Genetics

84–86. The answers are: 84-C, 85-B, 86-A. *(Gelehrter, pp 163–171. Thompson, 5/e, pp 201–214.)* Reciprocal translocations (diagram A) involve the exchange of segments between two chromosomes. Robertsonian translocations (diagram B) involve the joining of two acrocentric chromosomes by breakage and reunion of their short arms. Translocations that produce no duplication or deficiency are called *balanced.* Carriers of balanced translocations have normal phenotypes unless the translocation alters the expression of an important gene at the breakpoint region. Isochromosomes involve duplication of short (diagram C) or long (diagram E) arms, which produces perfectly metacentric chromosomes deficient in long- or short-arm material, respectively. Paracentric inversions (diagram D) alter the banding pattern but not the shape of the chromosome since they do not involve the centromere.

87–89. The answers are: 87-E, 88-B, 89-A. *(Gelehrter, pp 163–171. Thompson, 5/e, pp 201–214.)* The abbreviations *i* and *t* describe isochromosomes and translocation chromosomes, respectively. Isochromosomes create chromosomes with mirror-image duplication of the short or long arms (diagrams C and E). Reciprocal translocations (diagram A) involve exchange of segments between two chromosomes. A semicolon (;) indicates this exchange and is placed between the breakpoints. Robertsonian translocations join together two acrocentric chromosomes to form a metacentric chromosome (diagram B). Carriers of balanced reciprocal translocations have a normal chromosome number, while carriers of balanced Robertsonian translocations have only 45 chromosomes.

90–91. The answers are: 90-D, 91-A. *(Gelehrter, pp 159–192. Thompson, 5/e, pp 201–230.)* Meiosis is most easily understood by considering the sex chromosomes during spermatogenesis. Segregation of X and Y homologues occurs at meiosis I, followed by segregation of sister chromatids at meiosis II. Failure of segregation (i.e., nondisjunction) at meiosis I generates 24,XY and 22,O gametes, while nondisjunction at meiosis II generates 22,O and 24,XX or 24,YY gametes. (No sex chromosome is indicated by 22,O.) Thus, 47,XXY (Klinefelter syndrome) results from nondisjunction at meiosis I or II, while 47,XYY results only from nondisjunction at meiosis II. Two cell lines with different karyotypes imply mosaicism (e.g., Turner mosaicism—45,X/46,XX), unless the individual is a composite of cells from two zygotes (chimerism). Mosaicism occurs after fertilization by means of a correction of an abnormal karyotype or as a result of nondisjunction producing an abnormal cell line.

92–93. The answers are: 92-B, 93-A. *(Gelehrter, pp 159–192. Thompson, 5/e, pp 201–230.)* A chromosome number of 45, together with a 21/21 translocation, implies the absence of normal (untranslocated) 21 chromosomes in the patient. If an additional chromosome 21 were present, the chromosome number would be 46 and the patient would have Down syndrome. Patients with balanced Robertsonian translocations have increased risks for children with unbalanced karyotypes due to extra doses of the translocation chromosome. Mosaic Down syndrome patients have two cell lines (e.g., 46,XX/47XX+21).

94–96. The answers are: 94-B, 95-A, 96-E. *(Gelehrter, pp 159–192. Thompson, 5/e, pp 201–230.)* Barr bodies are the cytologic correlates of inactive X chromosomes. Dosage compensation in humans requires inactivation of all but one X chromosome in each cell so that males and females will have appropriate amounts of X chromosome gene products. Barr bodies or inactive X chromosomes will be one less than the total number of X chromosomes. Although the Barr body is visible as a dot near the inner side of the nuclear membrane in many somatic cells, tests to determine the number of Barr bodies (e.g., buccal smears) are no longer considered useful or reliable. Rapid determination of sex chromosome numbers (e.g., in infants with ambiguous external genitalia) can be performed by fluorescent in situ hybridization (FISH) analysis, using DNA probes for the X and Y chromosomes.

97–98. The answers are: 97-B, 98-C. *(Gelehrter, pp 159–192. Thompson, 5/e, pp 201–230.)* Carriers of balanced translocations or of inversions have risks for abnormal segregation and rearrangement of chromosomes at meiosis. The chromosomes align so as to maximize synapsis of homologous regions, but aberrant segregation or crossing over can then produce abnormal gametes. Diagram B shows the alignment of a Robertsonian translocation (e.g., between chromosomes 13 and 14) so as to maximize synapsis with the untranslocated chromosomes. Only segregation along lines 2 and 3 produces one normal and one balanced translocation gamete; other segregations (1,3 or 2,3) produce gametes with partial trisomy or monosomy. Alignment of chromosomes bearing reciprocal translocations is shown in diagram A, where segregation along line 1 produces unbalanced gametes. Diagrams C and D show alignment of paracentric or pericentric inversion chromosomes, respectively. Crossovers within inverted regions may produce duplications of chromosomes.

99–100. The answers are: 99-D, 100-C. *(Gelehrter, pp 159–192. Thompson, 5/e, pp 201–230.)* Interpretation of a karyotype begins with noting the sex chromosomes, then the number of autosomes, and finally any discrepancies between homologues in overall shape or banding pattern. In karyotype B, the XXY sex chromosomes and triple rather than paired autosomes indicates 3 × 23 = 69,XXY, while the single X chromosome in karyotype A indicates 45,X.

Karyotype C shows extra material (*arrow*) on one chromosome 14 homologue. This extra material has a similar shape and density to a chromosome 21, supporting the interpretation as 46,XY,t(14q21q). Karyotype D shows three copies of chromosome 21 that are typical of 47,XX+21.

101–102. The answers are: 101-C, 102-B. *(Gelehrter, pp 159–192. Thompson, 5/e, pp 201–230.)* Karyotype B indicates three copies of every autosome, while karyotype D has three copies only of chromosome 21 (trisomy 21 Down syndrome). The three copies of autosomes, two X chromosomes, and one Y chromosome in karyotype B indicates a 3n chromosome number consistent with triploidy. Such individuals have a lethal combination of growth delay and birth defects. Karyotype A shows monosomy X associated with Turner syndrome, while the 46,XY,t(14q21q) result in karyotype C is diagnostic of translocation Down syndrome.

103–107. The answers are: 103-B, 104-D, 105-E, 106-F, 107-H. *(Gelehrter, pp 159–192. Thompson, 5/e, pp 201–230.)* Chromosomes are routinely studied at mitotic metaphase where they consist of two sister chromatids joined at a centromere. The drawings in the question are idiograms that represent banded metaphase chromosomes after hypotonic treatment, spreading on slides, banding (H in diagram), and photomicroscopy. The short, or "petite," arm is positioned above the centromere (E in diagram) by convention and is represented by "p" (D in diagram). The long arm is called "q" merely because it is the next letter in the alphabet (F in diagram). Chromosomes are metacentric (A in diagram), submetacentric (B in diagram) or acrocentric (C in diagram), according to the relative lengths of the short arm. Acrocentric chromosomes have repetitive DNA at their tips, which forms satellites (G in diagram).

108–112. The answers are: 108-A, 109-G, 110-E, 111-F, 112-H. *(Gelehrter, pp 159–192. Thompson, 5/e, pp 201–230.)* The nomenclature 46,XY,del(4p) refers to deletion of a segment of undetermined length from the short arm of chromosome 4 (karyotype A, *arrow*). Shorthand terminology for this cytogenetic finding is 4p−, as employed to describe the 5p− deletion in karyotype E, the 18q− deletion in karyotype G, and the 13q− deletion in karyotype C. All are associated with clinical syndromes that may be described as the 13q− or 18q− syndromes. The terms 3q+ (karyotype F) and 14p+ (karyotype H) are less specific because they merely denote extra chromatin on the long arm of chromosome 3 or the short arm of chromosome 14. Identification of the source of this extra material requires either clinical correlation (e.g., probable 21 material if the patient had Down syndrome) or detailed banding and molecular studies. Karyotypes B and D have an extra sex chromosomes.

113–117. The answers are: 113-E, 114-F, 115-D, 116-B, 117-H. *(Gelehrter, pp 159–192. Thompson, 5/e, pp 201–230.)* The constellation of birth defects and an unusual appearance (syndromes) caused by chromosomal anomalies were often recognized before technology was available to demonstrate small deletions or duplications. Infants with a weak, cat-like cry were thought to have the cri du chat syndrome until the characteristic of chromosome 5 (5p− in karyotype E) was available for definitive diagnosis. Since most duplications or deletions of chromosomes are associated with a characteristic clinical syndrome, the patient's phenotype may be helpful in identifying extra chromosomal material. The banding pattern of the extra material on chromosome 3q in karyotype F suggests duplication of the 3q terminus, but definitive identification as dup(3q) requires either molecular studies or clinical correlation. The Klinefelter syndrome, which is characterized by small testes, sterility, gynecomastia (large breasts), and a tall, slim build in males, is associated with a 47,XXY karyotype (karyotype D). No name is associated with the 47,XYY syndrome (karyotype B), but controversial studies suggest an increased incidence in prison populations. The extra material on chromosome 14p (karyotype H) looks similar to chromosome 21, and knowledge that the patient has Down syndrome would confirm the identification as a 14/21 translocation.

118–122. The answers are: 118-B, 119-B, 120-D, 121-F, 122-G. *(Gelehrter, pp 19–23. Thompson, 5/e, pp 21–30.)* Diploid oogonia and spermatagonia (stage A) undergo two meiotic divisions that separate chromosomal homologues into haploid oocytes and sperm (stage J). At prophase of meiosis I, $4n$ copies of each chromosome are aligned in synapsis as tetrads (stage B). The first meiotic metaphase (stage C) aligns homologues for separation (no division of centromeres) (stage D), while the second meiotic metaphase (stage F) aligns chromosomes for separation of sister chromatids (stage G). Chiasmata (visible bridges between chromosomes) form at the tetrad stage and produce an average of one to two crossovers per chromosome to generate recombinant gametes (I).

123–127. The answers are: 123-A, 124-F, 125-F, 126-J, 127-J. *(Gelehrter, pp 19–23. Thompson, 5/e, pp 21–30.)* Primordial germ cells develop in the yolk sac and migrate to the embryonic gonad between 4 to 6 weeks of embryogenesis. Meiosis in females begins at about 5 months of fetal development with primary oocytes (stage A) entering prophase of meiosis division I. They remain suspended in prophase until puberty and ovulation, dividing into

secondary oocytes (stage F) and ova (stage J). At ovulation, the secondary
oocyte progresses to metaphase of meiosis II, then proceeds to become a mature ovum at the time of fertilization (with extrusion of the second polar
body). In males, meiosis begins at puberty with division of spermatogonia
(stage A) into secondary spermatocytes (stage B) and finally into sperm (stage
J). The ova and sperm are haploid gametes (stage J) that combine at fertilization to form diploid zygotes.

Mendelian Inheritance

DIRECTIONS: Each question below contains five suggested responses. Select the **one best** response to each question.

128. Autosomal recessive conditions are correctly characterized by which of the following statements?

(A) They are often associated with deficient enzyme activity
(B) Both alleles contain the same mutation
(C) They are more variable than autosomal dominant conditions
(D) Most persons do not carry any abnormal recessive genes
(E) Affected individuals are likely to have affected offspring

129. A man is affected with brachydactyly, an autosomal dominant trait that causes shortening of several fingers. What is the risk that the man's first child will have brachydactyly?

(A) 100 percent
(B) 75 percent
(C) 50 percent
(D) 25 percent
(E) Virtually 0

130. When reproductive fitness (f) is zero, the chance that the disorder is due to a new mutation is

(A) 0 percent
(B) 10 percent
(C) 25 percent
(D) 50 percent
(E) 100 percent

131. Ectrodactyly is an autosomal dominant trait that causes missing middle fingers (lobster-claw malformation). A grandfather and grandson both have ectrodactyly, but the intervening father has normal hands by x-ray. Which of the following terms would apply to this family?

(A) Incomplete penetrance
(B) New mutation
(C) Variable expressivity
(D) Germinal mosaicism
(E) Anticipation

Questions 132–135

A 4-year-old boy presents to the physician's office with coarse facies, short stature, stiffening of the joints, and mental retardation. Both parents, a 10-year-old sister and an 8-year-old brother all appear unaffected. The patient's mother is pregnant. She also had a brother who died at 15 years of age with similar findings that seemed to worsen with age. She also has a nephew (her sister's son) who exhibits similar features. You suspect a diagnosis of Hunter syndrome.

132. The most likely pattern of inheritance for this condition is

(A) autosomal dominant
(B) autosomal recessive
(C) X-linked dominant
(D) X-linked recessive
(E) none of the above

133. The risk that the fetus is affected is

(A) 100 percent
(B) 67 percent
(C) 50 percent
(D) 25 percent
(E) virtually 0

134. Amniocentesis is performed to determine the sex of the fetus. What is the risk that the child will be affected if the fetus is female?

(A) 100 percent
(B) 67 percent
(C) 50 percent
(D) 25 percent
(E) Virtually 0

135. What is the risk that the child will be affected if the fetus is male?

(A) 100 percent
(B) 67 percent
(C) 50 percent
(D) 25 percent
(E) Virtually 0

Questions 136–139

A couple comes to the physician's office after having had two sons affected with homocystinuria, a defect in cystathionine β-synthase. The first-born son is tall and thin, has dislocated lenses, and an IQ of 70. He has also had several episodes of deep venous thromboses. Because the diagnosis was made earlier in the second son and treatment with a special diet was initiated early, he is less severely affected. No other family members are affected. While taking a family history, the physician discovers that the parents are first cousins.

136. The most likely pattern of inheritance for this condition is
(A) autosomal dominant
(B) autosomal recessive
(C) X-linked dominant
(D) X-linked recessive
(E) none of the above

137. The risk that a third child to this couple would be affected with homocystinuria is
(A) 100 percent
(B) 67 percent
(C) 50 percent
(D) 25 percent
(E) virtually 0

138. Suppose that this couple has five children affected with homocystinuria. The risk that their sixth child will be affected is

(A) 100 percent
(B) 67 percent
(C) 50 percent
(D) 25 percent
(E) virtually 0

139. Although this disorder is potentially treatable, this couple is well aware of the burden of that treatment. They are, therefore, concerned that their sons may have children with homocystinuria. The risk that their affected son will have an affected child is

(A) 100 percent
(B) 67 percent
(C) 50 percent
(D) 25 percent
(E) virtually 0

Questions 140–142

Mr. Smith is affected with Crouzon syndrome. He is noted to have craniosynostosis (i.e., premature closure of the skull sutures), with unusual facies that include proptosis secondary to shallow orbits, hypoplasia of the maxilla, and a curved "parrot-like" nose. His son and brother are also affected, although two daughters and his wife are not.

140. The most likely pattern of inheritance of this disorder is

(A) autosomal dominant
(B) autosomal recessive
(C) X-linked dominant
(D) X-linked recessive
(E) none of the above

141. Mr. and Mrs. Smith are considering having another child. The physician counsels them that the risk that the child will be affected with Crouzon syndrome is

(A) 100 percent
(B) 67 percent
(C) 50 percent
(D) 25 percent
(E) virtually 0

142. Suppose that Mr. and Mrs. Smith had four affected and no unaffected children. The risk that another child will be affected with Crouzon syndrome is

(A) 100 percent
(B) 67 percent
(C) 50 percent
(D) 25 percent
(E) virtually 0

Questions 143–145

A patient presents to the physician's office to ask questions about color-blindness. The patient is color-blind as is one of his brothers. His maternal grandfather was color-blind, but his mother, father, daughter, and another brother are not.

143. The most likely mode of inheritance for color-blindness is

(A) autosomal dominant
(B) autosomal recessive
(C) X-linked dominant
(D) X-linked recessive
(E) none of the above

144. His daughter is now pregnant. The risk that her child will be color-blind is

(A) 100 percent
(B) 50 percent
(C) 25 percent
(D) 12.5 percent
(E) virtually 0

145. The patient's daughter gives birth to a son. The risk that the child is affected is now

(A) 100 percent
(B) 50 percent
(C) 25 percent
(D) 12.5 percent
(E) virtually 0

146. Little People of America (LPA) is a support group for individuals with short stature that conducts many workshops and social activities. Two individuals with achondroplasia, a common form of dwarfism, meet at a LPA convention and decide to marry and have children. What is their risk of having a child with this same autosomal dominant condition?

(A) 100 percent
(B) 75 percent
(C) 50 percent
(D) 25 percent
(E) Virtually 0

147. A woman with cystic fibrosis, an autosomal recessive condition, marries her first cousin. What is the risk that their first child will have cystic fibrosis?

(A) 1/2
(B) 1/4
(C) 1/8
(D) 1/16
(E) 1/32

148. A woman with no history of color-blindness marries a color-blind man. It is known that this form of color-blindness exhibits X-linked recessive inheritance. What are the risks for this couple of having a son or daughter who is color-blind?

(A) 100 percent
(B) 75 percent
(C) 50 percent
(D) 25 percent
(E) Virtually 0

149. A woman has a father with X-linked recessive color-blindness. She marries a normal man. What is the risk that their sons will be color-blind?

(A) 100 percent
(B) 75 percent
(C) 50 percent
(D) 25 percent
(E) Virtually 0

Questions 150–151

150. The pedigree below is best explained by which of the following inheritance patterns?

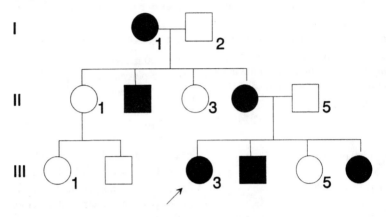

(A) Autosomal dominant inheritance
(B) Autosomal recessive inheritance
(C) X-linked recessive inheritance
(D) Polygenic inheritance
(E) Maternal inheritance

151. What would be the risk of individual III-3 having an affected child?

(A) 100 percent
(B) 75 percent
(C) 50 percent
(D) 25 percent
(E) Virtually 0

Questions 152–153

152. The pedigree below is best explained by which of the following inheritance patterns?

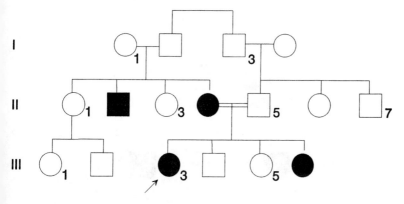

(A) Autosomal dominant inheritance
(B) Autosomal recessive inheritance
(C) X-linked recessive inheritance
(D) Autosomal dominant or autosomal recessive inheritance
(E) Maternal inheritance

153. What is the risk for individual II-2 of having an affected child if he mates with an unrelated woman?

(A) 100 percent
(B) 75 percent
(C) 50 percent
(D) 25 percent
(E) Virtually 0

Questions 154–155

154. The pedigree below is best explained by which of the following inheritance patterns?

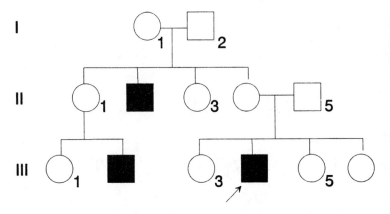

(A) Autosomal dominant inheritance
(B) Autosomal recessive inheritance
(C) X-linked recessive inheritance
(D) Autosomal dominant or autosomal recessive inheritance
(E) Maternal inheritance

155. What is the risk that a son born to individual III-3 would be affected?

(A) 100 percent
(B) 75 percent
(C) 50 percent
(D) 25 percent
(E) Virtually 0

Questions 156–157

156. The pedigree below is best explained by which of the following inheritance patterns?

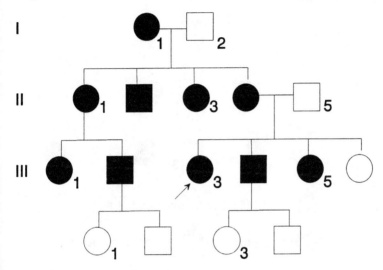

(A) Autosomal dominant inheritance
(B) Autosomal recessive inheritance
(C) X-linked recessive inheritance
(D) Autosomal dominant or autosomal recessive inheritance
(E) Maternal inheritance

157. The reason that individual III-6 is unaffected is because

(A) there is a 50:50 risk for transmission of abnormal mitochondrial alleles
(B) there are changes in the proportions of normal and abnormal mitochondria during embryogenesis
(C) a nuclear gene that interacts with the mitochondrial allele is likely
(D) individual III-6 is an example of a dispermic fertilization
(E) variable expressivity is present

Questions 158–159

It is known that cataracts, frontal baldness, myotonia (i.e., the inability to relax the muscles), and severe birth defects can all be caused by Steinert myotonic dystrophy, a Mendelian disorder.

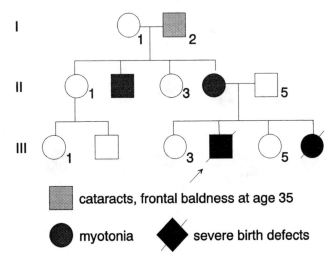

cataracts, frontal baldness at age 35

myotonia   severe birth defects

158. The pedigree above is most consistent with which of the following inheritance patterns?

(A) Autosomal dominant inheritance, incomplete penetrance
(B) Autosomal dominant inheritance, variable expressivity
(C) Autosomal dominant inheritance, new mutation
(D) Autosomal dominant inheritance, anticipation
(E) X-linked recessive inheritance

159. What would the risk be for individual II-2 of having a severely affected infant with lethal birth defects?

(A) 100 percent
(B) 75 percent
(C) 50 percent
(D) 25 percent
(E) Virtually 0

DIRECTIONS: Each numbered question or incomplete statement below is NEGATIVELY phrased. Select the **one best** lettered response.

160. All the following statements regarding autosomal dominant conditions are true EXCEPT

(A) they tend to have a vertical pattern in the pedigree
(B) men and women are equally affected
(C) the less the reproductive fitness, the less likely it is the case resulted from a new mutation
(D) they are often clinically variable
(E) they are pleiotropic

161. A man is identified as having an X-linked dominant disorder. His daughter appears unaffected. Possible explanations include all of the following EXCEPT

(A) Turner karyotype
(B) nonpaternity
(C) lyonization
(D) inheritance of unaffected paternal allele
(E) back mutation

162. X-linked recessive inheritance involves all the following factors EXCEPT

(A) oblique pattern of inheritance
(B) male-to-male transmission
(C) affected males and carrier females
(D) loci on the X chromosome
(E) new mutations for one-third of sporadic cases

163. An affected male infant born to normal parents could be an example of all the following disorders EXCEPT

(A) autosomal dominant disorder
(B) autosomal recessive disorder
(C) polygenic disorder
(D) vertically transmitted disorder
(E) X-linked recessive disorder

164. An individual who has one normal and one abnormal allele could transmit or be affected with all the following disorders EXCEPT

(A) autosomal dominant disorder
(B) X-linked dominant disorder
(C) autosomal recessive disorder
(D) X-linked recessive disorder
(E) homozygous disorder

165. Molecular genetic technology has demonstrated new mechanisms of inheritance that do not conform to simple Mendelian rules. Examples of atypical inheritance mechanisms include all the following EXCEPT

(A) mitochondrial inheritance
(B) genomic imprinting
(C) sporadic mutation
(D) trinucleotide repeat amplification
(E) maternal inheritance

166. Incontinentia pigmenti is a disorder that is lethal in utero in affected males. The findings may be very variable in females and include pigmented skin lesions, dental abnormalities, and patchy areas of alopecia. Some adults show only slightly atrophic depigmented areas. Approximately one-third of affected females have mental retardation. Approximately 45 percent of cases are the result of new mutations. All of the following statements regarding this disorder are true EXCEPT

(A) affected females show an increased frequency of spontaneous abortions
(B) the ratio of females to males in affected sibships is 3:1
(C) females have a 50 percent chance of inheriting the disorder from an affected mother
(D) the parents of affected individuals should be examined carefully
(E) unaffected males cannot transmit the phenotype

DIRECTIONS: Each group of questions below consists of lettered headings followed by a set of numbered items. For each numbered item select the **one** lettered heading with which it is **most** closely associated. Each lettered heading may be used **once, more than once or not at all.**

Questions 167–172

Match the descriptions that follow with the correct mode of inheritance?

(A) Autosomal dominant
(B) Autosomal recessive
(C) X-linked recessive
(D) Chromosomal
(E) Polygenic

167. Male-to-male transmission makes this mode unlikely

168. Elevated maternal age is characteristic

169. Parents with three affected children have a higher recurrence risk than parents with two affected children

170. Elevated paternal age is characteristic

171. Consanguinity is characteristic

172. Inborn errors of metabolism are associated

Questions 173–174

Match each of the numbered statements regarding X-linked inheritance below with the correct lettered statement.

(A) The disorder is genetically lethal in males
(B) The condition nearly always manifests itself in heterozygous females
(C) The condition is lethal in utero in hemizygous males
(D) Male-to-male transmission is possible
(E) Unaffected males transmit the phenotype

173. Approximately two-thirds of mothers of affected males are carriers

174. Women are affected twice as often as men

Questions 175–177

The pedigree below represents a family with retinitis pigmentosa, a genetically heterogeneous eye disease that causes progressive visual impairment. Match each of the individuals listed below with his or her risks.

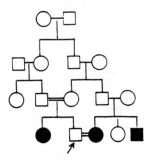

(A) 50 percent (1/2)
(B) 33 percent (1/3)
(C) 25 percent (1/4)
(D) 11 percent (1/9)
(E) Virtually 0

175. Risk for child of proband to have retinitis pigmentosa

176. Risk for parents of proband to have another child with retinitis pigmentosa

177. Risk for proband to have an affected child with retinitis pigmentosa if he had married his wife's unaffected sister

Questions 178–179

The pedigree below represents a family with retinitis pigmentosa. Match each of the individuals listed below with his or her risk.

(A) 50 percent (1/2)
(B) 33 percent (1/3)
(C) 25 percent (1/4)
(D) 11 percent (1/9)
(E) Virtually 0

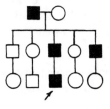

178. Risk for proband's son to have retinitis pigmentosa

179. Risk for proband's daughter to have retinitis pigmentosa

Questions 180–182

The pedigree below represents a family with retinosa pigmentosa. Match each of the individuals listed below with his or her risk.

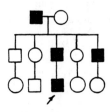

(A) 50 percent (1/2)
(B) 33 percent (1/3)
(C) 25 percent (1/4)
(D) 11 percent (1/9)
(E) Virtually 0

180. Risk for proband's son to have retinitis pigmentosa

181. Risk for proband's daughter to have retinitis pigmentosa

182. Risk for affected male's daughter to have a child with retinitis pigmentosa

Questions 183–185

For each case history that follows, select the term that best represents it.

(A) Allelic heterogeneity
(B) Locus heterogeneity
(C) Variable expressivity
(D) Incomplete penetrance
(E) New mutation

183. A grandson and paternal grandfather have ectrodactyly (i.e., an autosomal dominant disorder characterized by absent middle fingers), but the father has normal hands

184. An albino couple has a normal child (albinism is an autosomal recessive disorder)

185. A 90-year-old man with autosomal dominant neurofibromatosis has a son and grandson who died in their twenties from neural tumors

Questions 186–188

Match the terms below with the appropriate description.

(A) One locus, two identical alleles
(B) One locus, two different mutant alleles
(C) One locus, one normal allele, one mutant allele
(D) One locus, one allele
(E) Two loci, four different alleles

186. Heterozygote (carrier)

187. Compound heterozygote

188. Double heterozygote

Questions 189–191

Waardenburg syndrome is an autosomal condition that accounts for 1.4 percent of congenitally deaf individuals. In addition to deafness, patients with this condition have a typical facies, including lateral displacement of the inner canthi and partial albinism. Given that the mother has Waardenburg syndrome and the father is unaffected, match the number of affected children with the most likely probability.

(A) 1/8
(B) 1/4
(C) 3/8
(D) 1/3
(E) 1/2

189. None of three children affected

190. One of three children affected

191. Two of three children affected

Questions 192–194

The major blood group locus in humans produces types A (genotypes AA or AO), B (genotypes BB or BO), AB (genotype AB), or O (genotype OO). For each pair of parents, match the possible offspring.

(A) Type AB child
(B) Type B child
(C) Type O child
(D) None of above

192. Type O father, type AB mother

193. Type AB father, type O mother

194. Type A father, type A mother

Questions 195–197

Phenylketonuria (PKU) is an autosomal recessive disease that causes severe mental retardation if it is undetected. Two normal parents are told by their state neonatal screening program that their third child has PKU. Assuming that the initial screening is accurate, match each individual with the risk of having or being a carrier for PKU.

(A) 100 percent
(B) 67 percent
(C) 50 percent
(D) 25 percent
(E) Virtually 0

195. The risk of the next child having PKU

196. The risk of the eldest child being a carrier of PKU

197. The risk of the mother being a carrier of PKU

Questions 198–200

The pedigree below suggests a particular Mendelian inheritance pattern. Match the matings below with the risk of having an affected child.

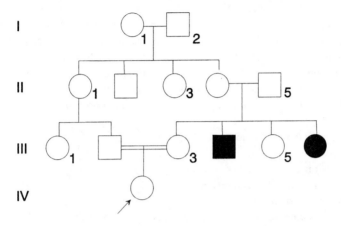

(A) 1/2
(B) 1/4
(C) 1/8
(D) 1/16
(E) 1/24

198. Individual III-1 mating with III-4

199. Individual III-2 mating with III-3

200. Individual II-5 with individual III-1

Questions 201–203

A couple presents for genetic counseling after their first child was born with achondroplasia (i.e., dwarfing syndrome). The physician obtains the following family history: The husband (George) is the first-born of four male children, and George's next oldest brother has cystic fibrosis. The wife is an only child. The couple and both sets of grandparents have had no remarkable medical problems.

The physician should now draw the pedigree with the female member of any couple on the left. The generations are numbered with Roman numerals and individuals with Arabic numerals; individuals affected with achondroplasia or cystic fibrosis are indicated. (Recall that achondroplasia is autosomal dominant and cystic fibrosis is autosomal recessive.) Match the individuals below with the appropriate description by referring to your numbered pedigree.

  (A) Affected with cystic fibrosis
  (B) Normal female
  (C) Normal male
  (D) Proband
  (E) Two-thirds chance of being a carrier of cystic fibrosis

201. Individual III-1

202. Individual I-1

203. Individual II-5

Questions 204–206

Achondroplasia is an autosomal dominant condition that is characterized by dwarfism, prominent forehead, shallow nasal bridge, and short limbs. Because of support groups such as Little People of America, achondroplasts often meet each other, marry, and have families. Match the probabilities below.

  (A) 100 percent
  (B) 75 percent
  (C) 50 percent
  (D) 25 percent
  (E) Virtually 0

204. The probability for the first child of achondroplastic parents to be affected (heterozygous or homozygous)

205. Following the birth of an affected child, the probability for the second child of acondroplastic parents to be affected

206. The probability for the first child to be affected if an achondroplast marries a normal person

Questions 207–209

Match the descriptions below with the appropriate risk figure.

(A) 100 percent
(B) 67 percent
(C) 50 percent
(D) 25 percent
(E) Virtually 0

207. The risk for a woman whose father has X-linked hemophilia to have an affected child

208. The risk for that same woman to have an affected son

209. The risk for a man with X-linked hemophilia to have an affected daughter

Questions 210–212

Tay-Sachs is an autosomal recessive disease that causes cherry-red spots in the eye, "startle" responses in infancy, neurodegeneration, and death. Heterozygotes with an abnormal Tay-Sachs allele are termed *carriers*. Match the following individuals with their risks to be carriers.

(A) 100 percent
(B) 67 percent
(C) 50 percent
(D) 25 percent
(E) Virtually 0

210. First cousin of an affected child

211. Grandmother of an affected child

212. Half-brother of an affected child

Questions 213–215

Two normal parents have a child with sensorineural deafness. Many genetic forms of deafness exist, including autosomal dominant, recessive, and X-linked forms. Match the following assumptions with the risk for a second affected child.

(A) 50 percent
(B) 50 percent or virtually 0
(C) 25 percent
(D) 25 percent or virtually 0
(E) Virtually 0

213. X-linked recessive inheritance

214. Autosomal dominant inheritance with complete penetrance

215. Autosomal dominant inheritance with incomplete penetrance

Questions 216–218

The pedigree shown in the figure below contains individuals with Charcot-Marie-Tooth (CMT) disease, a neurologic disorder that produces dysfunction of the distal extremities with characteristic footdrop. Match the individuals in the pedigree with their probability of having an affected child with CMT.

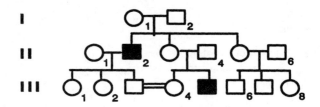

    (A) 1/2

    (B) 1/4

    (C) 1/8

    (D) 1/16

    (E) Virtually 0

216. Individual II-2

217. Individual II-3

218. Individual III-4

Questions 219–221

The pedigree shown in the figure below also contains individuals with Charcot-Marie Tooth (CMT) disease. However, this variant of CMT only becomes manifest in the late twenties. Match the individuals in the pedigree with their maximal risk of having an affected child with CMT given that III-8 and IV-1 through IV-9 are under age 25.

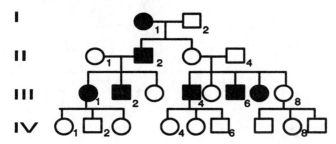

(A) 100 percent
(B) 50 percent
(C) 25 percent
(D) 12.5 percent
(E) Virtually 0

219. Individual II-3

220. Individual III-3

221. Individual IV-8

Questions 222–224

The pedigree in the figure below shows two members of a sibship affected with Charcot-Marie-Tooth (CMT) disease. Match the following individuals with the probability that their child will be affected. Assume that the incidence of this type of CMT in the general population is 1/10,000.

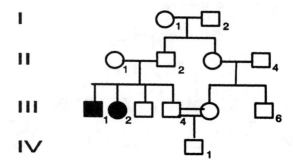

    (A) 1/24
    (B) 1/100
    (C) 1/300
    (D) 1/400
    (E) 1/800

222. Individual III-1

223. Individual III-3

224. Individuals III-4 or III-5

Questions 225–227

A woman who has two brothers with hemophilia A, an X-linked recessive disorder, and has had two normal sons is again pregnant. She requests counseling for the risk of her fetus to have hemophilia. Match the following risks.

    (A) 1
    (B) 1/2
    (C) 1/5
    (D) 1/10
    (E) 1/20

225. Risk for her mother to be a carrier

226. Risk for her to be a carrier if she had no children

227. Risk for her to be a carrier given two normal sons

Questions 228–230

The pedigree shown below shows a disease that causes early miscarriage or neonatal death of affected males and a normal life span in affected females. Based on the probable mode of inheritance, match the descriptions below with the probable risk figures.

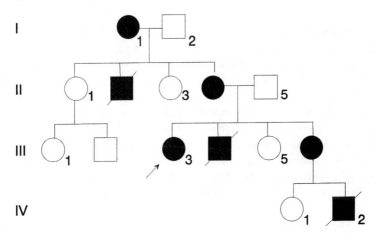

(A) 2/3
(B) 1/2
(C) 1/3
(D) 1/4
(E) Virtually 0

228. The risk that a son of individual III-3 will be affected with a lethal disease

229. The risk that a child of individual III-3 will be affected as an adult

230. The risk that a child of individual III-5 will be affected at any age

Mendelian Inheritance
Answers

128. The answer is A. *(Gelehrter, pp 36–39. Thompson, 5/e, pp 66–71.)* Autosomal recessive conditions tend to have a horizontal pattern in the pedigree. Men and women are affected with equal frequency and severity. It is the pattern of inheritance most often seen in cases of deficient enzyme activity (inborn errors of metabolism). Autosomal recessive conditions tend to be more severe than dominant conditions and are less variable than dominant phenotypes. Both alleles are defective but do not necessarily contain the exact same mutation. All individuals carry 6 to 12 mutant recessive alleles. Fortunately, most matings involve persons who have mutations at different loci. Since related persons are more likely to inherit the same mutant gene, consanguinity increases the possibility of homozygous affected offspring.

129. The answer is C. *(Gelehrter, pp 27–48. Thompson, 5/e, pp 53–96.)* The genotype of the man described in the question can be written as Bb, with the lower case b representing the abnormal brachydactyly allele. Assuming that the man's wife does not also have brachydactyly, her genotype can be represented as BB. The risk then depends on whether a B or b sperm fertilizes the egg, which is a risk of 50 percent.

130. The answer is E. *(Gelehrter, pp 39–44. Thompson, 5/e, pp 65–66.)* The fitness of a disorder (f) is a measure of the number of offspring born to affected persons in comparison to the number born to a control population. As the fitness is reduced and affected individuals have fewer children, the proportion of cases that arise as the result of new mutations increases. When $f = 0$—that is, when affected individuals do not reproduce—all new cases must be the result of a new mutation.

131. The answer is A. *(Gelehrter, pp 27–48. Thompson, 5/e, pp 143–166.)* *Incomplete penetrance* applies to a normal individual who is known from the pedigree to have an allele responsible for an autosomal dominant trait. *Variable expressivity* refers to family members who exhibit signs of the autosomal dominant disorder but vary in severity. When this severity seems to worsen with progressive generations, it is called *anticipation*. A new mutation in the grandson would be extremely unlikely given the affected grandfather.

The father could be an example of *somatic mosaicism* if a back mutation occurred in the cells that would form limb buds, but there is no reason to suspect mosaicism in his germ cells based on one affected son.

132–135. The answers are: 132-D, 133-D, 134-E, 135-C. *(Gelehrter, pp 39–44. Thompson, 5/e, pp 72–82.)* When evaluating the possibility of an X-linked disorder, it is important to remember the pattern of inheritance of the X chromosome. Females have two X chromosomes, which are passed along in a random fashion. They will pass any given X chromosome to 50 percent of their sons and 50 percent of their daughters. For a recessive condition, those daughters who inherit the affected allele will be heterozygous carriers of the disorder but will not be affected. Since males have only one X chromosome, those who inherit the affected allele will be affected with the disorder.

136–139. The answers are: 136-B, 137-D, 138-D, 139-E. *(Gelehrter, pp 36–39. Thompson, 5/e, pp 66–71.)* Autosomal recessive conditions tend to have a horizontal pattern in the pedigree. Although there may be multiple affected individuals within a sibship, parents, offspring, and other relatives are generally not affected. Most autosomal recessive conditions are rare; however, consanguinity greatly increases the likelihood that two individuals will have inherited the same mutant allele and pass it along to their offspring. The recurrence risk for an autosomal recessive condition is 1/4 or 25 percent. This risk is not affected by the genotype of the previous offspring. Since affected individuals must have two mutant alleles, they will pass an abnormal gene to all of their children. However, since these disorders are generally rare, it is unlikely that their partner will also carry a mutant allele at the same locus. Their children are virtually always heterozygous at this locus and phenotypically normal.

140–142. The answers are: 140-A, 141-C, 142-C. *(Gelehrter, pp 29–36. Thompson, 5/e, pp 59–66.)* In an autosomal dominant pedigree, there is a vertical pattern of inheritance. Assuming the disorder is not the result of a new mutation, every affected person has an affected parent. The same is true of X-linked dominant pedigrees. However, male-to-male transmission, as seen in this family, excludes the possibility of an X-linked disorder. A person with an autosomal dominant phenotype has one mutant allele and one normal allele. They randomly pass one or the other of these alleles to their offspring, giving a child a 50 percent chance of inheriting the mutant allele and, therefore, being affected with the disorder. This risk is unaffected by the genotype of the previous offspring.

143–145. The answers are: 143-D, 144-C, 145-D. *(Gelehrter, pp 39–44. Thompson, 5/e, pp 72–82.)* Males always transmit their single X chromosome to their daughters. Therefore, the female offspring of a male affected with an X-linked disorder is an obligate carrier for that disorder. When the condition is X-linked recessive, the daughter is unlikely to show any phenotypic evidence that she is carrying this abnormal gene. These female carriers may, in turn, pass along their genes in four different fashions: (1) mutant allele, female offspring, phenotype unaffected; (2) normal allele, female offspring, phenotype unaffected; (3) mutant allele, male offspring, phenotype affected; and (4) normal allele, male offspring, phenotype unaffected. Therefore, the chance of having an affected child is 1/4 or 25 percent. However, when only male offspring are considered the chance is 1/2 or 50 percent of having an affected child.

146. The answer is B. *(Gelehrter, pp 27–48. Thompson, 5/e, pp 53–96.)* The genotype of each dwarf can be represented as Aa, with the upper case A representing the achondroplasia allele. The Punnett square in the figure below demonstrates that 3/4 possible gamete combinations will yield individuals with at least one A allele. Homozygous AA achondroplasia is a severe disease that is particularly lethal in the newborn period.

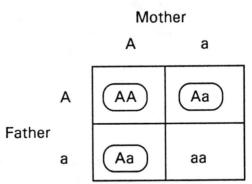

147. The answer is C. *(Gelehrter, pp 27–48. Thompson, 5/e, pp 53–96.)* The genotype of the affected woman with cystic fibrosis can be represented as the two lower case letters cc. Her parents are obligate carriers for the disorder (genotypes Cc), and one of her grandparents must also be a carrier (barring new mutations). Her first cousin then has a 1/4 chance of being a carrier, since one of their common grandparents is a carrier, one of his parents has a 1/2 chance of being a carrier, and he has a 1/2 chance of inheriting the c allele from his parent. The affected woman can only transmit c alleles to her fetus, while her cousin has 1/2 chance of transmitting his c allele if it is present.

Thus, the probability that the first child will have cystic fibrosis is 1/4 (cousin is carrier) $\times$ 1/2 (cousin transmits c allele) = 1/8 (fetus has cc genotype).

148. The answer is E. *(Gelehrter, pp 27–48. Thompson, 5/e, pp 53–96.)* The couple's daughters will be obligate carriers—that is, carriers implied by the pedigree. Representing the recessive color-blind allele by lower case c, the woman will be X^CX^C, while her husband will be X^cY. The Punnett square in the figure below indicates that all daughters will be X^CX^c while sons will be X^CY.

Mother

	X^C	X^C
X^c	X^CX^c	X^CX^c
Y	X^CY	X^CY

Father

Note again that loci on the X-chromosome cannot be transmitted from father to son, since the son receives the father's Y chromosome.

149. The answer is C. *(Gelehrter, pp 27–48. Thompson, 5/e, pp 53–96.)* The woman is an obligate carrier, since her father is color-blind. Her genotype can be represented as X^CX^c, while her normal husband's genotype is X^CY. Her sons can, thus, receive either the X^C or X^c alleles, making their risk of having color-blindness 50 percent. Her daughters will have a similar risk of being carriers.

150–151. The answers are: 150-A, 151-C. *(Gelehrter, pp 27–48. Thompson, 5/e, pp 53–96.)* Autosomal dominant inheritance is suggested by the pedigree that accompanies the question because of the vertical pattern of affected individuals and the affliction of both sexes. Autosomal recessive inheritance is ruled out by transmission through 3 generations, and X-linked recessive inheritance by the presence of affected females. Maternal inheritance should demonstrate transmission to all or most offspring of affected mothers. Polygenic or multifactorial inheritance is not associated with such a high frequency of transmission. Note that X-linked dominant inheritance would also be an explanation for the pedigree.

Because the most likely mechanism responsible for the pedigree is autosomal or X-linked dominant inheritance, individual III-3 is affected with the disorder, and she has a 50 percent risk of transmitting the disease. Discrimination between autosomal and X-linked dominant inheritance could be made by noting the offspring of affected males, such as individual III-4. If X-linked dominant inheritance were operative, affected males would have normal sons and affected daughters.

152–153. The answers are: 152-B, 153-E. *(Gelehrter, pp 27–48. Thompson, 5/e, pp 53–96.)* The presence of consanguinity *(double line in pedigree)* is a red flag for autosomal recessive inheritance because, although disease-causing alleles are rare, the probability of a homozygous individual escalates dramatically when the same rare allele descends through two branches of a family.

Carriers of autosomal recessive diseases are heterozygotes with one normal and one abnormal allele. Since most autosomal recessive diseases involve enzyme deficiencies, the carrier state indicates that 50 percent levels of enzymes are sufficient for normal function. If a carrier mates with an unrelated individual, the chance that that individual will also be a carrier is approximately twice the square root of the disease incidence. This figure derives from the Hardy-Weinberg law. Since most recessive diseases have incidences lower than 1/10,000, the risk for the unrelated mate to also be a carrier is less than 1/50, and the chance of having an affected child is less than $1/50 \times 1/4 =$ less than 1/200. Disorders such as cystic fibrosis that are fairly common in certain ethnic groups would be exceptions to this very low risk.

154–155. The answers are: 154-C, 155-D. *(Gelehrter, pp 27–48. Thompson, 5/e, pp 53–96.)* X-linked recessive inheritance is characterized by a predominance of affected males and an oblique pattern. Transmission must be through females with no evidence of male-to-male transmission. The lack of affected females would make autosomal dominant inheritance less likely, and the sex ratio plus transmission through 3 generations would eliminate autosomal recessive inheritance. Polygenic inheritance usually exhibits less frequent transmission, although it is certainly not ruled out in this pedigree. The many normal offspring of affected females rule out maternal inheritance.

Individual II-4 in the pedigree that accompanies the question is an obligate carrier since she has an affected brother and affected son. This means that her daughter (III-3) has a 1/2 chance of inheriting the X chromosome with an abnormal allele and 1/2 chance of inheriting the X chromosome with the normal allele. If individual III-3 is a carrier, she has a 1/2 chance of transmitting her abnormal allele to her son. The risk for her son to be affected is thus $1/2 \times 1/2 = 1/4$, or 25 percent. Since the daughters of individual III-3 might be carriers (1/2 chance) but will not be affected, individual III-3 has a 1/8 chance of having an affected child.

156–157. The answers are: 156-E, 157-B. *(Gelehrter, pp 27–48. Thompson, 5/e, pp 53–96.)* Nontraditional inheritance patterns have been increasingly appreciated as molecular technology allows direct examination of genes. Maternal inheritance is suggested by the pedigree that accompanies the question because affected women have affected offspring, while affected males do not. Autosomal dominant inheritance would be possible, but the ratio of affected to unaffected individuals would be unusually high compared to the expected 50:50 ratio. X-linked recessive inheritance is ruled out by the many affected females, and polygenic inheritance would not exhibit such high frequencies of transmission. A proven cause of maternal inheritance is mutation of mitochondrial DNA. Eggs contribute abundant cytoplasm that contains mitochondria, but sperm contribute little or none. Examples of mitochondrial diseases include a type of optic atrophy, muscular weakness–epilepsy syndromes, and even certain forms of diabetes mellitus.

Because there can be as many as 1000 mitochondria per cell, changes in the proportion of normal versus abnormal mitochondrial DNAs can change during cell division. This means that individuals are frequently mosaic for the proportions of abnormal and normal mitochondria in different tissues, a condition called *heteroplasmy*. Females have many hundreds of mitochondrial alleles in their eggs, not just two. Fertilization of an egg by two sperm produces triploidy, not a fetus with male-derived mitochondria. Zygotes formed by fusion of two sperm pronuclei have been produced in mice, and they do not survive past early embryogenesis. Variable expressivity refers to variable expression among family members with an autosomal dominant disorder. Nuclear interaction with mitochondrial alleles does occur, but correction of a mitochondrial disorder by nuclear alleles is unlikely.

158–159. The answers are: 158-D, 159-E. *(Gelehrter, pp 29–48. Thompson, 5/e, pp 53–96.)* Anticipation refers to the worsening of the symptoms of disease in succeeding generations. The famous geneticist L. S. Penrose dismissed anticipation as an artifact, but the phenomenon has been validated by the discovery of expanding trinucleotide repeats. Steinert myotonic dystrophy is caused by unstable trinucleotide repeats near a muscle protein kinase gene on chromosome 19; the repeats are particularly unstable during female meiosis and may cause a severe syndrome of fetal muscle weakness and joint contractures as in individuals III-4 and III-6. Variable expressivity could also be used to describe the pedigree, but the concept implies random variation in severity rather than progression with succeeding generations. X-linked recessive inheritance is ruled out by the instances of male-to-male transmission (I-2 to II-2).

Affected males with myotonic dystrophy (individual II-2) have a low risk for dramatic triplet repeat expansion in their offspring so as to completely ablate muscle protein kinase expression and produce a severely affected offspring. Individual II-2 would have a 50 percent risk for an affected child, but triplet repeat instability seems to be exaggerated during meiosis in affected females. Diseases that involve triplet repeat instability exhibit a bias for exaggerated repeat amplification during meiosis (e.g., women with the fragile X syndrome and myotonic dystrophy and men with Huntington's chorea). The explanation for this bias is unknown.

160. The answer is C. *(Gelehrter, pp 29–36. Thompson, 5/e, pp 59–66.)* Autosomal dominant conditions tend to have a vertical pattern in the pedigree. (See pedigree in the figure that accompanies questions 178–179.) Men and women are affected with equal frequency and severity. The frequency of isolated cases (presumably due to a new mutation) increases with the severity of the disorder; that is, the lesser the reproductive fitness, the more likely it is to have resulted from a new mutation. Autosomal dominant conditions are generally clinically variable and pleiotropic (i.e., have multiple phenotypic features that frequently appear to be unrelated).

161. The answer is D. *(Gelehrter, pp 39–44. Thompson, 5/e, pp 74–82.)* In an X-linked dominant disorder, affected males transmit their single, affected X chromosome to all their daughters. The unaffected chromosome is the Y chromosome, which is transmitted to all sons. In the Turner (XO) phenotype, females have only one X chromosome and, therefore, may not have inherited the affected allele. In some cases, favorable lyonization results in the inactivation of the majority of X chromosomes that bear the affected allele. Back mutation may result in the reappearance of the normal allele. Nonpaternity would also explain the lack of inheritance of the abnormal phenotype.

162. The answer is B. *(Gelehrter, pp 27–48. Thompson, 5/e, pp 53–96.)* Loci on the X chromosome cannot be transmitted from father to son, since the son receives the father's Y chromosome. X-linked recessive disorders do display oblique patterns of inheritance with sisters of affected males transmitting mutant alleles to their sons. Because women have two X chromosomes, they are unaffected with X-linked recessive disorders except in rare cases of nonrandom lyonization or X-autosomal translocations. For sporadic cases—that is, cases without a family history—the chance that the mother is a carrier is 2/3 and that her son represents a new mutation is 1/3. This rule was deduced by J. B. S. Haldane and is based on the fact that the mother has two X chromosomes that could be the site of a mutation, while her son has one.

163. The answer is D. *(Gelehrter, pp 27–48. Thompson, 5/e, pp 53–96.)* The most common dilemma in genetic counseling is an index case without any family history. It is important to realize that the proband could represent a new mutation for an X-linked or autosomal dominant disorder, a new mutation (if male) for an X-linked recessive disorder, or an inherited disorder from parents who are carriers for autosomal or X-linked recessive traits. Chromosomal disorders may also arise de novo from balanced translocation carriers, and polygenic disorders can arise from parents who are shifted towards but not across the threshold of expression. Vertical transmission—that is, parental-child transmission—provides suggestive evidence for a genetic etiology, but infectious diseases, maternal diseases that affect the developing fetus, and other environmental causes may mimic genetic transmission. For these reasons, interpretation of a sporadic case is entirely dependent on the diagnosis.

164. The answer is E. *(Gelehrter, pp 27–48. Thompson, 5/e, pp 53–96.)* Mechanisms of inheritance are properties of gene action rather than of the gene itself. It is incorrect to refer to an "autosomal dominant gene" because it is the type of gene action that determines expression of the trait. Heterozygotes may be completely normal if the mutant allele encodes an enzyme (i.e., autosomal recessive inheritance) or even structural components that are compensated by genetic background (i.e., autosomal dominant inheritance, variable expressivity). Hypercholesterolemia is usually considered an autosomal dominant disorder in which one mutant allele causes a predisposition to heart attacks. In primitive societies with high-fiber diets and short life spans, only homozygotes with two defective alleles encoding the low-density lipoprotein (LDL) receptor would have sufficiently high cholesterols to have symptoms. In these primitive societies, hypercholesterolemia would be considered a rare autosomal recessive disease.

165. The answer is C. *(Gelehrter, pp 27–48. Thompson, 5/e, pp 53–96.)* The possibility of new mutations to explain the occurrence of isolated (sporadic) cases has long been recognized for autosomal dominant or X-linked recessive disorders. Higher rates of mutation were approximately one mutation per 10^4 individuals per generation. Trinucleotide repeat amplification provided a new mechanism for mutation with unprecedented rates up to one mutation per individual per generation. Genomic imprinting involves "marking" of genes differently when inherited through sperm or eggs.

166. The answer is B. *(Gelehrter, pp 39–44. Thompson, 5/e, pp 79–82.)* The fact that a disorder is lethal in utero in males does not alter the normal sex ratios for conception. Women who are affected with such conditions still conceive 50 percent males and 50 percent females. One-half of the males inherit the affected X chromosome, and those pregnancies will end in spontaneous abortion. Since the disorder does not affect the in utero viability of females, twice as many females as males are born. Additionally, since all males who survive to term must be unaffected and, therefore, have inherited the normal allele, they cannot pass the disorder to their offspring. In disorders such as this one where affected individuals may have only very mild manifestations, it is crucial to examine the parents of affected individuals very carefully to determine if the mutant allele has been inherited or is the result of a new mutation.

167–172. The answers are: 167-C, 168-D, 169-E, 170-A, 171-B, 172-B. *(Gelehrter, pp 27–48. Thompson, 5/e, pp 53–86.)* Males must transmit their Y chromosome to produce sons, which rules out the possibility for male-to-male transmission of X chromosome alleles. Elevated maternal age is associated with an increased risk for chromosomal nondisjunction. Maternal age over 35 is considered an indication for amniocentesis. An increasing recurrence risk according to the number of relatives affected is characteristic of polygenic inheritance. The more affected relatives, the more evidence there is that an individual's genetic background is shifted towards the threshold for a particular trait; for example, the expectation for tall parents with tall grandparents is to have tall children.

Elevated paternal age is associated with increased risk for new mutations. Since autosomal dominant traits require only one abnormal allele for expression, it is autosomal dominant disorders that frequently present as new mutations. Autosomal recessive inheritance is the rule for inborn errors of metabolism since many are enzyme deficiencies. The presence of one normal allele (50 percent of normal enzyme levels) is usually sufficient to prevent disease. Consanguinity should raise suspicion of autosomal recessive traits because the same rare allele may become homozygous in a consanguineous individual.

173–174. The answers are: 173-A, 174-B. *(Gelehrter, pp 39–44. Thompson, 5/e, pp 72–82.)* In X-linked inheritance, no male-to-male transmission of the phenotype occurs, and unaffected males do not transmit the phenotype. When the disorder is genetically lethal in males (i.e., the affected male does not reproduce), approximately one-third of cases arise as the result of a new mutation; the remaining two-thirds have heterozygous carrier mothers who generally are unaffected. This phenomenon is known as the *Haldane hypothesis*. When the disorder is nearly always manifest in females, there will be about twice as many affected females as males (since they have twice the chance of receiving an X chromosome).

175–177. The answers are: 175-B, 176-C, 177-D. *(Gelehrter, pp 27–47. Thompson, 5/e, pp 53–88.)* In the pedigree that accompanies the question, there is a horizontal pattern of inheritance typical of autosomal recessive disorders. This inheritance pattern is also supported by the presence of consanguinity. The proband has a 2/3 chance of being a carrier, and the consanguinity suggests that his wife is homozygous for the same retinitis pigmentosa alleles. The risk is thus $2/3 \times 1/2$ for the proband to contribute the recessive allele, while his wife has a 100 percent chance to do so, which results in a final probability of 1/3 that the child will be affected. This decreases to 1/9 if the proband marries his wife's unaffected sister, who also has a 2/3 chance of being a carrier.

178–179. The answers are: 178-A, 179-A. *(Gelehrter, pp 27–47. Thompson, 5/e, pp 53–88.)* The pedigree that accompanies the question has the vertical pattern suggestive of autosomal dominant inheritance. Although all affected individuals are male, X-linked inheritance is ruled out by the instance of male-to-male transmission. Affected individuals have a 50 percent chance of having affected offspring, regardless of sex.

180–182. The answers are: 180-C, 181-E, 182-C. *(Gelehrter, pp 27–47. Thompson, 5/e, pp 53–88.)* The pedigree that accompanies the question has the oblique pattern of X-linked recessive inheritance. The proband has a 1/2 chance of being a carrier, and thus, each of her sons has a 1/4 chance of being affected; however, overall there is a 1/8 chance of an affected child since 1/2 of her children will be male. Unless there is nonrandom lyonization of the X chromosome that carries the normal retinitis pigmentosa allele, female carriers should not be affected. X-linked inheritance implies that affected males cannot transmit diseases to their sons and that their daughters will be obligate carriers.

183–185. The answers are: 183-D, 184-B, 185-C. *(Gelehrter, pp 27–45. Thompson, 5/e, pp 53–95.)* Autosomal dominant disorders often vary in severity within families (variable expressivity) but occasionally are clinically silent in a person known to carry the abnormal allele (incomplete penetrance). Albinism is one of many genetic diseases that exhibit locus heterogeneity, which means that mutations at several different loci can produce identical phenotypes.

186–188. The answers are: 186-C, 187-B, 188-E. *(Gelehrter, p 27. Thompson, 5/e, pp 53–54.)* A heterozygote or, in the case of an autosomal recessive disorder, a carrier, has one normal allele and one mutant allele at a given locus. A compound heterozygote has two different mutant alleles, and a double heterozygote has one mutant allele at each of two different loci.

189–191. The answers are: 189-A, 190-C, 191-C. *(Gelehrter, pp 30–31. Thompson, 5/e, pp 146–147.)* For each pregnancy, the probability that the child will be affected is 1/2. Therefore, the probability that all three children will be affected is the product of the three independent events—that is, $1/2 \times 1/2 \times 1/2 = 1/8$. The probability that all three children will be unaffected is the same. When evaluating the probability that one of the three children will be affected, it must be noted that there are three of eight possible birth orders that have one affected child (Www, wWw, wwW). The probability of two affected children is also 3/8. In general, the probability of any given number of affected children can be determined by using the binomial expansion, $(p + q)^n$, where p and q are the probabilities of two alternative events $(1 - p = q)$, and n is the number of events. In this case, $p = 1/2$, $q = 1/2$, and $(p + q)^3 = p^3 + 3p^2q + 3pq^2 + q^3$.

$$p_3 = 1/8 = \text{probability of three unaffected}$$
$$3p^2q = 3/8 = \text{probability of two unaffectded, one affected}$$
$$3pq^2 = 3/8 = \text{probability of one unaffected, two affected}$$
$$q^3 = 1/8 = \text{probability of three affected}$$

192–194. The answers are: 192-B, 193-B, 194-C. *(Gelehrter, pp 27–47. Thompson, 5/e, pp 53–88.)* Diploid persons have two alleles per autosomal locus with one being transmitted to each gamete (Mendel's law of segregation). The key to blood group problems is to recognize that a blood type is ambiguous regarding possible alleles—type A persons may have AA or AO genotypes. Once the possible genotypes are deduced from the blood types, potential offspring will represent all combinations of parental alleles.

195–197. The answers are: 195-D, 196-B, 197-A. *(Gelehrter, pp 36–39. Thompson, 5/e, pp 66–72.)* If the abnormal allele is represented as p and the normal as P, an infant affected with phenylketonuria (PKU) will have the genotype pp. Parents must be heterozygotes or carriers (Pp) for the child to inherit the p allele from both the mother and father (assuming correct paternity and the absence of unusual chromosomal segregation). Subsequent children have a 1/2 chance of inheriting allele p from the mother and a 1/2 chance of inheriting allele p from the father; the chance that both events will occur to give genotype pp is thus $1/2 \times 1/2 = 1/4$, or 25 percent. A normal sibling may be genotype PP (1/4 probability) or Pp (1/2 probability since two different combinations of parental alleles give this genotype). The ratio of these probabilities results in a 2/3 chance (67 percent) of genotype Pp (note that genotype pp is excluded because a normal sibling was specified).

198–200. The answers are: 198-C, 199-E, 200-D. *(Gelehrter, pp 27–48. Thompson, 5/e, pp 53–96.)* The pedigree that accompanies the question suggests autosomal recessive inheritance because of the affected brother and sister. The consanguineous mating is incidental rather than causal. Individual III-1 has an aunt (individual II-4) who must be a carrier, since she has two affected children. This means one grandparent (I-1 or I-2) must be a carrier with a 1/2 chance that II-1 is a carrier and a 1/2 chance that III-1 inherited the abnormal allele from her mother II-1. Individual III-1 has a $1/2 \times 1/2 = 1/4$ chance to be a carrier, while individual III-4 is homozygous affected and can only transmit an abnormal allele. If III-1 is a carrier, she has a 1/2 chance of transmitting her abnormal allele, resulting in a final risk of 1/8 for an affected child. A similar calculation applies to individual III-2, yielding a 1/4 risk to be a carrier, while III-3 has a 2/3 chance to be a carrier because of her affected siblings. The final risk is $1/4 \times 2/3 \times 1/4 = 1/24$ that their next child will be affected. Since II-5 is an obligate carrier, his mating with III-1 would have a $1/4 \times 1/4 = 1/16$ risk for an affected child.

201–203. The answers are: 201-D, 202-B, 203-E. *(Gelehrter, pp 27–47. Thompson, 5/e, pp 53–88.)* The figure below shows the correctly drawn pedigree with generations indicated by Roman numerals and individuals by Arabic numbers.

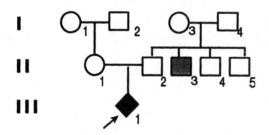

The person who prompted genetic concern is the proband (III-1). Individual II-5, like George, has a brother with cystic fibrosis. Since the parents (I-3, I-4) are carriers, the brother had a 1/4 chance of being normal, a 2/4 chance of being a carrier, and a 1/4 chance of being affected with cystic fibrosis. If the possibility of being affected is eliminated (as given in the pedigree), the odds of being a carrier are 2/3.

204–206. The answers are: 204-B, 205-B, 206-C. *(Gelehrter, pp 36–39. Thompson, 5/e, pp 66–72.)* Representing the abnormal allele as A and the normal as a, achondroplastic parents (Aa) will produce AA, Aa, and aa children with respective probabilities of 1/4, 2/4, and 1/4. Since both AA and Aa children will be affected with achondroplasia, the total risk is 3/4 (75 percent) for an achondroplastic child. Chance has no memory, so the same risk applies for each pregnancy regardless of prior outcomes. If an achondroplast (Aa) and normal person (aa) marry, their risk is 50 percent to have a child with achondroplastic dwarfism (Aa). The homozygous individual with achondroplasia (genotype AA) is in fact more severely affected and often dies in the newborn period.

207–209. The answers are: 207-D, 208-C, 209-E. *(Gelehrter, pp 39–45. Thompson, 5/e, pp 74–83.)* Women have two X chromosomes; men an X chromosome and a Y chromosome. X-linked inheritance implies that the abnormal allele resides on the X chromosome. Males have one allele that is either normal or abnormal (hemizygosity), while women will usually be homozygous normal or heterozygous (carriers). Rarely, women may be homozygous abnormal. Female offspring of affected males must receive their father's X to be female; they are, thus, obligate carriers of the abnormal allele. Carrier females have a 25 percent chance to have affected children or a 50 percent chance if the offspring is male. Affected males cannot transmit the disease to sons because, by definition, they have transmitted their Y rather than their X chromosome.

210–212. The answers are: 210-D, 211-C, 212-C. *(Gelehrter, pp 36–39. Thompson, 5/e, pp 66–72.)* Parents of children with autosomal recessive disorders are obligate carriers if nonpaternity and rare examples of uniparental disomy (inheritance of chromosomal homologues from the same parent) are excluded. Normal siblings have a 2/3 chance to be carriers since they cannot be homozygous for the abnormal allele. Grandparents have a 1/2 chance to be carriers because one or the other of them must have transmitted the abnormal allele to the obligate carrier parent. First cousins share a set of grandparents of whom one must be a carrier. There is a 1/2 chance for the aunt or uncle to be a carrier and 1/4 chance for the first cousin. Half-siblings share an obligate carrier parent and have a 1/2 chance to be carriers. These calculations assume the lack of mutations (Tay-Sachs is rare) and the lack of coincidental alleles (no consanguinity).

213–215. The answers are: 213-D, 214-E, 215-B. *(Gelehrter, pp 27–45. Thompson, 5/e, pp 53–95.)* Parents of a child affected with an autosomal recessive disease are usually carriers with a 1/4 risk of having a second affected child. If a son is affected with an X-linked disease, the mother may be a carrier (1/4 risk for subsequent children) or not (virtually 0 risk). Children affected with autosomal dominant diseases either represent a new mutation (neither parent affected with virtually 0 recurrence risk) or inherit their abnormal allele from a parent (50 percent recurrence risk). If the parents are phenotypically normal, they will have virtually 0 recurrence risk unless one has the abnormal allele (incomplete penetrance). In the latter case, their recurrence risk is 50 percent. For X-linked dominant inheritance, the affected male or female may represent a new mutation (virtually 0 recurrence risk) or transmission from an affected mother (50 percent recurrence risk).

216–218. The answers are: 216-E, 217-B, 218-C. *(Gelehrter, pp 39–44. Thompson, 5/e, pp 72–82.)* The predominance of affected males with transmission through females makes this pedigree diagnostic of X-linked recessive inheritance. Individual I-1 is an obligate carrier as demonstrated by her affected son and grandson. Individual II-2 cannot transmit an X-linked disorder, although his daughters are obligate carriers. Individual II-3 must be a carrier because of her affected son, which results in a 1/4 probability for recurrence of CMT in her offspring. Individual II-5 has a 1/2 probability of being a carrier with a 1/8 probability for affected offspring. Individual III-4 also has a 1/2 probability of being a carrier; her risk for affected offspring is also 1/8 despite the consanguineous marriage. Individual III-8 has a 1/4 chance of being a carrier and a 1/16 chance of having affected offspring.

219–221. The answers are: 219-B, 220-E, 221-D. *(Gelehrter, pp 29–36. Thompson, 5/e, pp 59–66.)* The vertical inheritance pattern (multiple affected generations) and equal sex ratio is suggestive of autosomal dominant inheritance for this form of Charcot-Marie-Tooth (CMT) disease. Individual III-1 is affected and has a 50 percent recurrence risk in each offspring. Individual II-3 is most likely an example of incomplete penetrance since she has three affected children. Individual III-3 is old enough to show the disease but is not affected and, thus, has a virtually 0 recurrence risk (excluding the possibility of incomplete penetrance). Individual III-8 is not old enough to manifest CMT and, therefore, has a maximal 50 percent chance of having the abnormal allele with a maximal 25 percent chance for affected children. Her daughter (individual IV-8), thus, has a maximal 12.5 percent chance that her child will be affected.

222–224. The answers are: 222-B, 223-C, 224-A. *(Gelehrter, pp 36–39. Thompson, 5/e, pp 66–72.)* Affected siblings of different sexes suggest autosomal recessive inheritance. Individual III-1 will, thus, be homozygous for the abnormal Charcot-Marie-Tooth (CMT) allele, while the probability that his future wife will be a carrier is twice the square root of the population incidence ($2pq$ from the Hardy-Weinberg law = $2 \times 1 \times 100$). The probability that his child will be affected is thus $1/50 \times 1/2 = 1/100$. Similarly, individual III-3 has a 2/3 chance of being a carrier and a 1/300 chance that his child will be affected. Individual III-4 has a 2/3 chance of being a carrier, and III-5 a 1/4 chance based on their common grandparents. The chance their second child will be affected is $2/3 \times 1/4 \times 1/4 = 1/24$. Individual III-6 also has a 1/4 chance to be a carrier, and the chance that his child will be affected is $1/4 \times 1/50 \times 1/4 = 1/800$. For II-3, her chance of being a carrier is 1/2, the chance for an unrelated husband to be a carrier 1/50, and the final probability for an affected child is $1/2 \times 1/50 \times 1/4 = 1/400$.

225–227. The answers are: 225-A, 226-B, 227-C. *(Gelehrter, pp 264–267. Thompson, 5/e, pp 400–409.)* Since the consultand's mother has two affected sons with hemophilia, she is an obligate carrier (excluding rare instances of germinal mosaicism). Her daughter has a 1/2 chance to receive the X that carries the abnormal gene. However, the fact that the daughter has two normal boys can be taken into account by using Bayes theorem. The easiest way to do this is to set up a table as shown below:

	Woman Is Carrier	**Not Carrier**
Prior probability	1/2	1/2
Conditional (given 2 normal boys)	1/4	1
Joint (prior × conditional)	1/8	4/8
Adjusted probability	$\dfrac{1/8}{1/8 + 4/8} = 1/5$	$\dfrac{4/8}{1/8 + 4/8} = 4/5$

Given a 1/5 chance to be a carrier, the woman's risk for an affected child is $1/5 \times 1/4 = 1/20$ (1/10 for a male to be affected).

228–230. The answers are: 228-B, 229-C, 230-E. *(Gelehrter, pp 27–48. Thompson, 5/e, pp 53–96.)* The pedigree demonstrates transmission through females with approximately equal numbers of offspring being affected. This is characteristic of X-linked dominant inheritance. Several disorders, including incontinentia pigmenti, orofaciodigital syndrome, and Goltz syndrome, exhibit lethality in affected males due to their single X chromosome. In many cases, the affected males present as early miscarriages, so that only affected females are recognized. Affected females have a 50 percent risk that their sons will be affected, and 1/3 chance for an affected older child (the possibilities are normal daughter, affected daughter, and normal son with affected sons not surviving to birth). Unaffected females do not have the abnormal allele and, thus, have no risk for affected children.

Population Genetics and Polygenic Inheritance

DIRECTIONS: Each question below contains five suggested responses. Select the **one best** response to each question.

231. In a population in which random mating occurs, 50 percent of the people in 1 generation have the genotype Aa. In the following generation, the percentage of people with genotype Aa will be

(A) 100 percent
(B) 75 percent
(C) 50 percent
(D) 25 percent
(E) 0 percent

232. A guanidine thymidine (GT) polymorphism has five different possible alleles, each with a frequency of 0.2. The percentage of people who are heterozygous is

(A) 20 percent
(B) 40 percent
(C) 50 percent
(D) 60 percent
(E) 80 percent

233. Galactosemia is an inborn error of metabolism in which infants present with failure to thrive, vomiting, jaundice, hepatomegaly, and cataracts. The frequency of this disorder is approximately 1/40,000 live births (0.000025). The frequency of the carrier state is approximately

(A) 0.02
(B) 0.01
(C) 0.005
(D) 0.002
(E) 0.001

234. For recessive diseases, the Hardy-Weinberg term $p^2 + 2pq + q^2$ provides the explanation for three important phenomena. First, elimination of homozygous abnormal individuals does not significantly decrease the incidence of the disease. Second, an advantage for heterozygous carriers may have a dramatic effect in increasing the incidence of a recessive disease. Third, parental consanguinity should alert the physician to the possibility of recessive disease in offspring. Recalling that q is usually employed for the frequency of abnormal alleles in recessive disorders, select the explanation of these phenomena.

(A) $q^2 > p^2$
(B) $2pq > p^2$
(C) $q^2 > 2pq$ and $2pq > p^2$
(D) $p^2 > 2pq > q^2$
(E) $p^2 > q^2$

235. Isolated cleft lip and palate is a multifactorial trait. The recurrence risk of isolated cleft lip and palate is

(A) the same in all families
(B) not dependent upon the number of affected family members
(C) the same in all ethnic groups
(D) the same in males and females
(E) affected by the severity of the cleft

236. Achondroplasia is an autosomal dominant form of skeletal dysplasia that produces dwarfism. Rarely, two affected individuals (heterozygotes) mate and produce a severely affected homozygote. Representing the abnormal allele frequency by p and the normal allele frequency by q, why does the Hardy-Weinberg law predict that homozygotes will be rare in dominant diseases?

(A) Affected individuals, represented by the genotype frequency q^2, will be very rare
(B) Affected individuals, represented by the genotype frequency p^2, will be very rare
(C) The genotype frequency $2pq$, which represents affected heterozygotes, will be much larger than p^2, which represents affected homozygotes
(D) Assortative mating is rare because achondroplasts do not meet
(E) Achondroplasia in homozygotes is prenatally lethal

237. Achondroplasts have about 80 percent less viable offspring than do normal persons. This has certain implications for the mutation rate since the incidence of achondroplasia is thought to have remained constant for some time. Representing fitness by f, the coefficient of selection by s, and the mutation rate by μ, a true statement is

(A) s is 0.8, f is 0.2, μ is relatively high

(B) s is 0.4, f is 0.2, μ is relatively low

(C) s is 0.2, f is 0.8, μ is relatively high

(D) s is 0.2, f is 0.2, μ is relatively high

(E) s is 0.2, f is 0.8, μ is relatively low

238. Many disorders that present in adult life, such as coronary artery disease and hypertension, are multifactorial traits. A multifactorial trait results from

(A) the interaction between the environment and a single gene

(B) the interaction between the environment and multiple genes

(C) multiple postnatal environmental factors

(D) multiple pre- and postnatal environmental factors

(E) multiple genes independent of environmental factors

Questions 239–241

A newborn boy dies with severe hyperammonemia. Prior to his death, a diagnosis was made of ornithine transcarbamylase (OTC) deficiency, an X-linked disorder of urea cycle metabolism, which in its classic form is lethal in males. Answer the following questions with regard to this family.

239. The likelihood that the proband's disease is the result of a new mutation is

(A) 100 percent

(B) 67 percent

(C) 50 percent

(D) 33 percent

(E) 25 percent

240. Subsequent testing reveals that the proband's mother is a carrier of the disease. The chance that her next child will be affected is

(A) 67 percent

(B) 50 percent

(C) 33 percent

(D) 25 percent

(E) 0 percent

241. The proband's mother remarries. The chance that her next child will be affected is

(A) 67 percent

(B) 50 percent

(C) 33 percent

(D) 25 percent

(E) 0 percent

242. In a certain population, 4 percent of individuals have homozygous aa genotypes for a polymorphic locus with alleles A and a. What are the allele frequencies for A and a?

(A) A = 0.9; a = 0.2
(B) A = 0.8; a = 0.2
(C) A = 0.7; a = 0.2
(D) A = 0.8; a = 0.04
(E) A = 0.96; a = 0.04

243. A polymorphic locus has alleles A and a that are tested in sperm and found to have frequencies of 90 percent and 10 percent, respectively, for the pooled sperm from a population bank. If white blood cells are now tested in this population of 100, how many individuals are expected to be AB heterozygotes?

(A) 99
(B) 81
(C) 36
(D) 18
(E) 9

244. A certain birth defect occurs with 1/2 probability if an individual is simultaneously heterozygous for the rare polymorphic alleles at four different loci. Each locus has two alleles Aa, Bb, Cc, Dd with the lower case alleles being the rarer of the two. Survey of the population shows that heterozygotes at any one locus average 10 percent. The probable incidence of the birth defect in the population is

(A) 1/100
(B) 1/1000
(C) 1/200
(D) 1/2000
(E) 1/20,000

DIRECTIONS: Each numbered question or incomplete statement below is NEGATIVELY phrased. Select the **one best** lettered response.

245. All the following statements regarding twins are true EXCEPT

(A) the frequency of monozygotic twins is greater than the frequency of dizygotic twins

(B) the frequency of twin births is different in different ethnic groups

(C) among North American Caucasians, the incidence of twinning is approximately 1/87 live births

(D) monozygotic twins may be mono- or dichorionic

(E) 50 percent of dizygotic twin pairs are same sex

246. A polymorphic locus has three alleles Q, R, and S with approximately equal population frequencies. Which of the following factors is LEAST likely to cause a change in these frequencies?

(A) A selective advantage for SS individuals in finding food

(B) A preference of QS individuals to mate with RS or SS individuals

(C) A doubling of the population size

(D) Migration of SS individuals into the population

(E) Extinction of all but a few individuals in the population among normal individuals

247. All the following characteristics are typical of polymorphic loci EXCEPT

(A) a variable DNA restriction site produces a large restriction fragment upon Southern blotting in 2 percent of individuals

(B) starch gel electrophoresis demonstrates variant mobility of the haptoglobin protein in 10 percent of individuals

(C) DNA sequencing reveals an A/T substitution in 8 percent of introns separating β-globin gene exons

(D) catalase enzyme has subunits of different size

(E) a dinucleotide CA sequence exhibits between 5 and 15 repeats among normal individuals

248. All the following assumptions must be valid for the Hardy-Weinberg equilibrium to apply to allele frequencies in a population EXCEPT

(A) no selection

(B) random mating

(C) no mutation

(D) no expansion

(E) no migration

Questions 249–251

Random mating assumes that there is no stratification, assortative mating, or consanguinity.

249. All the following statements regarding assortative mating are true EXCEPT

(A) the choice of mate is influenced by the traits that mate possesses
(B) it increases the percentage of homozygous genotypes
(C) the expectations of the Hardy-Weinberg equation do not necessarily apply
(D) long-term population effects are great
(E) the families involved may have a high genetic risk

250. All the following statements regarding stratification are true EXCEPT

(A) population subgroups are largely genetically distinct
(B) it increases the percentage of homozygous genotypes
(C) few stratified populations exist
(D) different subgroups have different incidences of specific diseases
(E) different subgroups have different mutant alleles

251. All the following statements regarding consanguinity are true EXCEPT

(A) it increases the percentage of heterozygous genotypes
(B) the rarer the disorder, the more likely that consanguinity is present
(C) it is commoner in certain populations
(D) intermarriage of third cousins is genetically insignificant
(E) most matings are at least remotely consanguineous

DIRECTIONS: Each group of questions below consists of lettered headings followed by a set of numbered items. For each numbered item select the **one** lettered heading with which it is **most** closely associated. Each lettered heading may be used **once, more than once or not at all.**

Questions 252–254

Match the terms listed below with the appropriate partial definitions.

(A) Gradual diffusion of genes between populations
(B) Proportion of genes that are identical by descent
(C) All genes present at a given locus
(D) Random fluctuation of genes in small populations
(E) Complete DNA sequence of an organism

252. Gene pool

253. Genetic drift

254. Gene flow

Questions 255–257

Match each of the ethnic groups listed below with the genetic disorder commonly associated with it.

(A) Cystic fibrosis
(B) Beta Thalassemias
(C) Tay-Sachs disease
(D) Down syndrome
(E) Sickle cell anemia

255. African Americans

256. Greek Americans

257. Jewish Americans

Questions 258–260

Match each of the following statements about allele frequency with the term that best describes it.

(A) Selection for allele A
(B) Linkage disequilibrium with allele A
(C) Linkage to allele A
(D) Founder effect for allele A
(E) Assortative mating for allele A

258. A study of diabetes mellitus patients shows that 82 percent have AA or Aa genotypes

259. The ship Hopewell arrived on a small island several hundred years ago, carrying numerous pilgrims with diabetes insipidus. This disease is now known to be caused by mutant allele A, and residents of the island have 10 times the frequency of this allele as do those on the mainland

260. A family study shows that the paternal grandfather, six of his children, and 12 grandchildren all have allele A along with cataracts

Questions 261–262

Match the following situations with the appropriate terms.

(A) Founder effect
(B) Heterozygote advantage
(C) Genetic lethal
(D) Fitness
(E) Natural selection

261. Increased resistance to malaria is seen in persons with hemoglobin AS, where A is the normal allele and S is the allele for sickle hemoglobin

262. There is a high frequency among the Amish of Ellis-van Creveld syndrome, an autosomal recessive disorder characterized by short-limbed dwarfism, polydactyly, hypoplastic nails, and cardiac defects. The Amish in this country are descendants of a small religious isolate who do not marry outside their sect

Questions 263–264

In a population in Hardy-Weinberg equilibrium in which 16 percent of the people have genotype AA, match the following genotypes listed below with their percentage of the population, assuming that a and A are the only alleles possible.

(A) 16 percent
(B) 24 percent
(C) 36 percent
(D) 48 percent
(E) 84 percent

263. Genotype aa

264. Genotype Aa

Questions 265–266

DNA analysis of a two-allele polymorphism (A, a) is performed on a large population of unrelated individuals. Twenty-five percent of people are found to be homozygous (AA). Match the alleles below with their probable frequencies.

(A) 0.125
(B) 0.25
(C) 0.5
(D) 0.625
(E) 0.75

265. A allele

266. a allele

Questions 267–269

Assume that frequencies for the different blood group alleles are as follows: A = 0.3; B = 0.1; O = 0.6. Match the blood types listed below with the percentage of people expected to have those blood types.

(A) 7 percent
(B) 13 percent
(C) 27 percent
(D) 36 percent
(E) 45 percent

267. Blood type A

268. Blood type B

269. Blood type O

Questions 270–272

A blood bank wishes to estimate donor availability in their area but does not have the resources for an extensive survey. Using United States averages for the frequency of MN blood group alleles, the blood bank predicts the number of available donors, assuming Hardy-Weinberg equilibrium. Based on frequencies for the M allele of 0.6 and N allele of 0.4, match the individuals described below with the estimates of donor availability per 1000 individuals.

(A) 1000
(B) 480
(C) 360
(D) 240
(E) 160

270. Type M individual

271. Type MN individual

272. Donors for type MN recipients

Questions 273–275

Match the following pairs of related individuals with their proportion of genes in common.

(A) One
(B) One-half
(C) One-fourth
(D) One-eighth
(E) One-sixteenth

273. Brother and sister

274. Parent and child

275. Brother and half sister

Questions 276–278

Tay-Sachs disease is a recessive degenerative neurologic disorder. The frequency of Tay-Sachs carriers among Ashkenazi Jews is 1/30. The frequency of Tay-Sachs carriers among Caucasians of Western European descent is approximately 1/300. Using this information, match the unions listed below with the chance that a child of that union will have Tay-Sachs disease.

(A) 1/120
(B) 1/240
(C) 1/3600
(D) 1/9000
(E) 1/36,000

276. Both parents are Ashkenazi Jews

277. The mother has an affected child by a previous union; the father is an Ashkenazi Jew

278. The mother is an Ashkenazi Jew; the father is a Caucasian from Western Europe

Questions 279–281

For each clinical situation listed below, select the probability figure that applies to it.

(A) 1/8
(B) 1/16
(C) 1/60
(D) 1/120
(E) 1/256

279. A man whose brother has cystic fibrosis wants to know his risk of having an affected child; the prevalence of cystic fibrosis is 1 in 1600 individuals

280. An African-American couple with a normal family history wants to know their chance of having a child with sickle cell anemia; the incidence of sickle cell trait is 1 in 8 for African Americans

281. A woman who married her first cousin wants to know the risk of having a child with cystic fibrosis because her grandmother who is also her husband's grandmother died of cystic fibrosis

Questions 282–284

Many common birth defects, such as cleft palate or myelomeningocele, follow the polygenic, or multifactorial, inheritance model with threshold. This model attempts to explain the following empirical risks that a relative faces if there is an affected person in the family: identical twin, 20 to 40 percent; first-degree relative, 2 to 3 percent; two first-degree relatives, 4 to 6 percent; three first-degree relatives, 6 to 9 percent; and second-degree relatives, 0.5 percent. Based on these figures, match the individuals below with their appropriate risk.

(A) 20 to 40 percent
(B) 6 to 9 percent
(C) 4 to 6 percent
(D) 2 to 3 percent
(E) 0.5 percent

282. Twin brother of a girl with congenital dislocated hip

283. Sibling of two children with a congenital heart defect and an affected parent

284. Grandchild of a person with spina bifida

Questions 285–287

Based on frequencies of 0.7 for allele O, 0.2 for allele A, 0.1 for allele B, 0.6 for allele M, and 0.4 for allele N in a population sample, match the indicated blood types with their expected number per 1000 people. The ABO and MN blood group loci are not linked.

(A) 490
(B) 154
(C) 150
(D) 40
(E) 24

285. Type O

286. Type B

287. Type B, N

Population Genetics and Polygenic Inheritance

Answers

231. The answer is C. *(Gelehrter, pp 49–52. Thompson, 5/e, pp 143–152.)* When random mating occurs, the frequency of genotypes remains constant over time. Therefore, if the frequency of the genotype Aa is 50 percent in 1 generation, it will remain 50 percent in subsequent generations. This situation is known as *Hardy-Weinberg equilibrium.*

232. The answer is E. *(Gelehrter, pp 146–147. Thompson, 5/e, pp 143–152.)* For each allele, the frequency of homozygotes is $(0.2)^2$. Therefore, the total number of homozygotes in this five-allele system is $5(0.2)^2$, or 0.2. The frequency of heterozygotes is $1 -$ (homozygotes), or 0.8. The answer can also be calculated using the binomial expansion $(p + q)^5$.

233. The answer is B. *(Gelehrter, pp 49–52. Thompson, 5/e, pp 145–153.)* The Hardy-Weinberg expansion, $p^2 + 2pq + q^2$, describes the frequency of genotypes for allele frequencies p and q. In the case of rare disorders ($q^2 < 0.0001$), p approaches 1. The heterozygote frequency $2pq$ is, thus, approximately $2q$. In this case, $q^2 = 0.000025$, $q = 0.005$, and $2q = 0.01$.

234. The answer is D. *(Gelehrter, pp 49–65. Thompson, 5/e, pp 143–165.)* In a recessive disease, most abnormal alleles reside in carriers since $p > q$ and $p^2 > 2pq > q^2$. For example, a disorder of incidence 1/10,000 (quite common for a recessive disease) will have $q = 1/100$, $p = 99/100$, and $2pq = 1/50$. In a population of 10 million, there will be 9.8 million normal individuals, 200,000 carriers, and 1000 affected individuals for this disease locus (assuming minimal selection). Eliminating the 1000 affected individuals will, thus, do little to affect the 200,000 abnormal alleles in carriers, but biologic or political factors that encourage carrier reproduction will have a 200-fold greater impact on abnormal allele frequency than measures that enhance homozygote survival. Since carriers are still quite rare compared with normal individuals, the matching of rare recessive alleles is greatly enhanced when there is common descent through consanguinity.

235. The answer is E. *(Gelehrter, pp 57–65. Thompson, 5/e, pp 349–363.)* Cleft lip with or without cleft palate [CL(P)]is one of the most common congenital malformations. Because of the genetic component of this trait, it tends to be more common in certain families. The more family members affected and the more severe the cleft, the higher the recurrence risk. In addition, CL(P) is more common in males and in certain ethnic groups (i.e., Asians > Caucasians > African Americans).

236. The answer is C. *(Gelehrter, pp 49–65. Thompson, 5/e, pp 143–165.)* The Hardy-Weinberg term $p^2 + 2pq + q^2$ is useful for considering relative frequencies of genotypes even though these will be modified slightly by selection, migration, or inbreeding in actual populations. Since the incidence of achondroplasia is less than 1 in 10,000 births, the frequency of the abnormal allele (usually p is taken as the abnormal allele frequency in dominant diseases) is quite small (q is approximately equal to 1). For this reason, $p^2 < 2pq < q^2$, and homozygous abnormal patients will be extremely rare for most dominant diseases. Assortative mating (preferential mating among certain genotypes) is not uncommon in achondroplasia because of activities sponsored by organizations such as Little People of America. Such matings are the main source of homozygotes.

237. The answer is A. *(Gelehrter, pp 49–65. Thompson, 5/e, pp 143–165.)* If an abnormal allele is as likely to be transmitted to the next generation as its corresponding normal allele, it is said to have a fitness (f) of 1. Loss of fitness (decrease in allele frequency after 1 generation) is measured by the coefficient of selection (s) where $f = 1 - s$. If achondroplasts have only 1/5 of the children of parents of normal stature in the population, then their fitness is 0.2 and the coefficient of selection is 0.8. The achondroplast alleles eliminated by selection must be replaced by mutation if the disorder has not disappeared or declined in incidence. Thus the mutation rate (μ) would be expected to be high relative to more benign dominant diseases.

238. The answer is B. *(Gelehrter, pp 57–65. Thompson, 5/e, pp 349–363.)* Many common disorders tend to run in families but are not single-gene or chromosomal disorders. These disorders are multifactorial traits, which are caused by multiple genetic and environmental factors. The term *polygenic* refers to those disorders that result from the interaction of multiple genes with no obvious environmental component.

239–241. The answers are: 239-D, 240-D, 241-D. *(Gelehrter, pp 39–44. Thompson, 5/e, pp 72–82, 163.)* For X-linked lethal disorders, two-thirds of the cases result from an abnormal gene passed on by a carrier mother, and one-third of cases result from a new mutation. This rule is known as the Haldane hypothesis and is named for J. B. S. Haldane who first described it in

1935. A woman who is a carrier of an X-linked lethal disorder passes that gene on to half her children with the following results: 1/4 carrier daughters, 1/4 affected sons, and 1/2 unaffected children. Since this is an X-linked disorder, these proportions are not dependent on the father in any way and will not change if the mother remarries.

242. The answer is B. *(Gelehrter, pp 49–68. Thompson, 5/e, pp 143–166.)* Allele frequencies in populations can be calculated using the Hardy-Weinberg equilibrium. If the frequency of allele A is designated as p, and the frequency of allele a is q, than $p + q = 1$ for a locus with only two alleles. The genotype frequencies are given by the expansion of this term, $p^2 + 2pq + q^2 = 1$, where p^2 represents AA homozygotes, $2pq$ the Aa heterozygotes, and q^2 the aa homozygotes. Since the frequency of aa homozygotes in this population is 0.04, the allele frequency of a = 0.2 and that of A = 0.8.

243. The answer is D. *(Gelehrter, pp 49–68. Thompson, 5/e, pp 143–166.)* Since gametes are haploid and have one allele per locus, the frequency of alleles A and a in pooled sperm should equal their population frequency. For diploid cells from that same population, the probability of the first allele being A is 0.9 and of the second allele being B is 0.1. The joint probability for a genotype of AB is thus $0.9 \times 0.1 = 0.09$. However, heterozygotes also can have a genotype of BA, so the added probabilities of AB or BA is 0.18. Of 100 individuals, 18 would be expected to be heterozygotes.

244. The answer is E. *(Gelehrter, pp 49–68. Thompson, 5/e, pp 143–166.)* The question mimics the multifactorial inheritance/threshold model for many common birth defects and predicts a chance for heterozygosity at all four loci of $0.1 \times 0.1 \times 0.1 \times 0.1 = 1/10,000$. Since the heterozygous fetus has a 1/2 chance to develop the birth defect, the birth incidence should be 1/20,000. This 1/2 probability represents the environmental contribution to many birth defects, in this case combining with the four rarer alleles to cross a threshold from normal to abnormal structure.

245. The answer is A. *(Thompson, 5/e, pp 389–391.)* Twins may be either monozygotic (identical) or dizygotic (fraternal). Monozygotic twins arise from a single zygote, which divides during early embryonic development. Depending on the timing of that division, monozygotic twins may be mono- or diamniotic and mono- or dichorionic. Dizygotic twins arise from two different zygotes and are diamniotic and dichorionic. The frequency of monozygotic twins is the same in all populations (i.e., approximately 1 in 260 live births), whereas the frequency of dizygotic twins is different in different populations. The frequency of any type of twinning among North American

Caucasians is about 1/87 live births. All monozygotic twins and 50 percent of dizygotic twins are same sex.

246. The answer is C. *(Gelehrter, pp 49–68. Thompson, 5/e, pp 143–166.)* Doubling of a population does not change allele frequencies (often referred to as gene frequencies) unless the initial population is very small. A small group has a greater chance to transmit an unusual distribution of alleles, just as a few coin flips may give all heads or tails rather than equal proportions. This effect is called *genetic drift*, and it may exaggerate the frequency and persistence of a mutant allele if it is present in the founder population (*founder effect*). Mating according to genotype or its phenotypic effects is called *assortative mating*, and it enhances the frequency of the preferred alleles in the next generation. Environmental circumstances that favor certain alleles (*selection*) also enhance their frequency; selection is thought to be the most important mechanism for evolution.

247. The answer is D. *(Gelehrter, pp 52–55. Thompson, 5/e, pp 143–166.)* Polymorphic loci have two or more alleles with the rarest maintaining a frequency greater than expected by new mutation. In practice, this means a frequency of greater than 1 percent for the rarest allele. Polymorphisms may be detected at the gene sequence level (variable numbers of nucleotide repeats, altered DNA restriction sites) or at the protein level (altered migration on electrophoretic gels, altered enzyme activity). Polymorphisms usually are harmless variations; alleles that cause disease are more often called mutations; for example, mutant alleles cause cystic fibrosis or sickle cell anemia. Multiple subunit proteins are not examples of polymorphism; they may be multimers of a single-gene product or aggregates of multiple-gene products. Cellular and morphologic phenotypes may also be described as polymorphic (i.e., fingerprints), but these are usually determined by multiple loci plus the environment (multifactorial traits).

248. The answer is D. *(Gelehrter, pp 49–65. Thompson, 5/e, pp 143–165.)* For a single locus with alleles M and N, the frequency of allele M can be represented by p and that of allele N by q. Obviously, $p + q = 1$. Under certain conditions, as pointed out independently by Hardy and Weinberg, the proportion of individuals with genotypes MM, MN, and NN will derive from the expansion $(p + q)(p + q) = p^2 + 2pq + q^2$. If the frequency of M is 0.9 and that of N is 0.1, then the proportion of MM (0.81), MN (0.18), and NN (0.01) individuals would be predicted. Note that these proportions ($p^2 + 2pq + q^2$) must also add up to 1. If, however, the measured proportions were 0.9 for MM, 0.1 for MN, and virtually 0 for NN, then there would be deviation from the Hardy-Weinberg law. Such discrepancies occur when there is selection (e.g., lethality of genotype NN), migration, or nonrandom mating (e.g., mutual aversion of MN heterozygotes). Population expansion could occur without altering the Hardy-Weinberg equilibrium.

249–251. The answers are: 249-D, 250-C, 251-A. *(Gelehrter, pp 49–57. Thompson, 5/e, pp 150–152.)* Assortative mating is the selection of a mate because of the specific traits of that mate. It is, by definition, nonrandom mating. Although it may be positive or negative, it is most common for individuals to select mates who resemble them in some fashion, including ethnicity, religion, or shared talents or interests. When these traits are genetically determined, the frequency of homozygosity increases. When individuals with similar mutant alleles, such as those for deafness or neuromuscular disease, mate, the expectations of the Hardy-Weinberg equation may no longer hold true because there is not a random distribution of genotypes. Although the genetic consequences may be great for the families involved, the consequences for the population as a whole are insignificant. It is interesting to consider the effect that support groups and social organizations that bring together individuals with similar disorders may have in promoting assortative mating.

Consanguinity brings together individuals who share an increased proportion of alleles, which are identical by descent. As a result, the percentage of homozygosity also increases. When alleles are uncommon, it is more likely that homozygosity results from consanguinity. Although closely consanguineous relationships are both illegal and morally taboo in most areas of the United States, they are common in certain populations. Some degree of consanguinity is quite common, however, as any two individuals are likely to have at least one ancestor in common if one goes back far enough. Matings between individuals who are third cousins or more remotely related tend not to be genetically significant.

Stratification is the phenomenon in which subgroups within populations remain genetically distinct. In the United States, for example, intermarriage between races or religions is relatively uncommon. As a result, there tends to be an increased frequency of homozygosity in these subgroups. Additionally, specific disorders and specific mutant alleles are more or less common in these subgroups than in the population as a whole.

252–254. The answers are: 252-C, 253-D, 254-A. *(Gelehrter, pp 143–165. Thompson, 5/e, pp 49–57.)* The *gene pool* is the total of all the alleles at a particular locus for the entire population. When calculating allele frequencies, a small cross section of the population is evaluated and generalizations are drawn. It is crucial that this cross section be representative of the entire population or estimates of gene (or allele) frequencies will be incorrect.

Genetic drift refers to the random fluctuations that are seen in gene frequencies over time. These fluctuations occur more often in small populations. They are the result of both new mutations and the isolation of small subpopulations.

Gene flow, on the other hand, is the slow diffusion of genes from one population to another. This results from migration and intermating.

The total DNA sequence of an organism is referred to as the *genome.* The proportion of genes that are identical by descent is the coefficient of relationship (*r*).

255–257. The answers are: 255-E, 256-B, 257-C. *(Gelehrter, pp 49–68. Thompson, 5/e, pp 143–166.)* Allele frequencies may differ among populations when there has been geographic isolation, founder effects, or selection for certain alleles based on different environments. Although African Americans have intermixed with Caucasians in the United States for over 400 years, they retain a higher frequency of sickle cell alleles, which are thought to protect individuals from malarial infection. Each ethnic group has frequencies of polymorphic alleles that reflect its origin; for example, Ashkenazi Jews have a higher frequency of Tay-Sachs alleles; Greeks and other Mediterranean peoples, thalassemia alleles; and Caucasians, cystic fibrosis alleles. Down syndrome, a chromosomal disorder, has virtually the same frequency of 1 in 600 births among all ethnic groups. The preservation of genetic differences after migration allows the use of highly polymorphic mitochondrial genes to trace relationships among ancient and modern human populations.

258–260. The answers are: 258-B, 259-D, 260-C. *(Gelehrter, pp 49–68. Thompson, 5/e, pp 143–166.)* Linkage disequilibrium describes an association between a particular polymorphic allele and a trait. Many autoimmune diseases exhibit association with particular human leukocyte antigen (HLA) alleles (i.e., HLA-B27 and ankylosing spondylitis). The association is not necessarily cause and effect (e.g., when viral infections that trigger a disease preferentially infect certain HLA genotypes).

Founder effects represent a special case of genetic drift in which rare alleles are introduced into a small population by the migration of ancestors.

Genetic linkage implies physical proximity of the allele locus to the gene causing the disease. Linkage differs from allele association in that either allele A or a may be linked in a given family, depending on which allele is present together with the offending gene.

Neither assortative mating (preferential mating by genotype) or selection (advantageous alleles) applies to the examples in the questions.

261–262. The answers are: 261-B, 262-A. *(Gelehrter, pp 49–55. Thompson, 5/e, pp 143–166.)* Sickle cell anemia is the classic example of a disorder with a high frequency in a specific population because of *heterozygote advantage*. Persons who are heterozygous for this mutant allele (hemoglobin AS) have increased resistance to malaria and are, therefore, at an advantage in areas where malaria is endemic.

Founder effect is a special type of genetic drift. In these cases, the founder or original ancestor of a population has a certain mutant allele. Because of genetic isolation and inbreeding, that allele is maintained at a relatively high frequency. There is also a high frequency of certain diseases caused by the homozygosity of alleles, which are identical by descent.

Fitness is a measure of the ability to reproduce. A *genetic lethal* implies that affected individuals cannot reproduce and, therefore, cannot pass on their mutant alleles. *Natural selection* is a theory introduced by Charles Darwin, which postulates that the fittest individuals have a selective advantage for survival.

263–264. The answers are: 263-C, 264-D. *(Gelehrter, pp 49–52. Thompson, 5/e, pp 143–152.)* The Hardy-Weinberg equation states that the proportion of individuals with a given genotype in a two-allele system can be determined from the binomial expression $(p + q)^2$, where p and q are the frequencies of the two alleles and $p + q = 1$. The frequencies of the genotypes are p^2, $2pq$, and q^2. In this case, AA or $p^2 = 0.16$, and A $= 0.4$. Since A $+$ a $= 1$, a $= 0.6$ and aa or $q^2 = 0.36$. The frequency of Aa is $2pq$ or $2 \times 0.4 \times 0.6 = 0.48$. Please note that $0.16 + 0.48 + 0.36 = 1$.

265–266. The answers are: 265-C, 266-C. *(Gelehrter, pp 49–52. Thompson, 5/e, pp 143–152.)* Using the Hardy-Weinberg expansion, $p^2 + 2pq + q^2$, p^2 is 0.25 and p, or the frequency of the A allele, is 0.5. Since $1 - p = q$, q is also 0.5.

267–269. The answers are: 267-E, 268-B, 269-D. *(Gelehrter, pp 49–52. Thompson, 5/e, pp 121–123, 145–149.)* It is important to remember that individuals with blood type A can have either genotype AA or AO, and individuals with blood type B can have either genotype BB or BO. Therefore, the frequency of blood type A is the frequency of homozygotes—that is, 0.3×0.3—plus the frequency of heterozygotes—that is, $2(0.3) \times 0.6$—for a total of 0.45. The frequency of blood type B is $0.1 \times 0.1 + 2(0.1) \times 0.6$ for a total of 0.13. The frequency of individuals with blood type O is simply the frequency of homozygotes—that is, $0.6 \times 0.6 = 0.36$.

270–272. The answers are: 270-C, 271-B, 272-A. *(Gelehrter, pp 49–65. Thompson, 5/e, pp 143–165.)* Allele frequencies provide a simple and direct way of estimating the frequency of genotypes in the population if the Hardy-Weinberg equilibrium applies. Assigning the higher frequency of allele M as

p and the lower frequency of allele N as q, then genotype frequencies are MM (p^2) = 0.6 × 2 = 0.36; MN $(2pq)$ = 2 × 0.6 × 0.4 = 0.48; and NN (q^2) = 0.4 × 2 = 0.24. Since MN individuals have acquired tolerance to both the M and N antigens on their red cells, they are universal recipients with regard to the MN blood group (100 percent of the population).

273–275. The answers are: 273-B, 274-B, 275-C. *(Gelehrter, pp 52–59. Thompson, 5/e, pp 152–155.)* Although all individuals, other than identical twins, are genetically unique, we all share some genes in common with our relatives. The more closely we are related, the more genes we have in common. First-degree relatives, such as siblings, parents, and children, share one-half of their genes. Second-degree relatives share one-fourth, and third-degree relatives share one-eighth.

276–278. The answers are: 276-C, 277-A, 278-E. *(Gelehrter, pp 30–31, 49–52. Thompson, 5/e, pp 143–152.)* To determine the joint probability of two or more independent events, the product of their separate probabilities must be determined. The parents who are both Ashkenazi Jews have a 1/30 chance of carrying an abnormal gene for Tay-Sachs disease; for each pregnancy, they have a 1/2 chance of passing that gene along should they carry it. The probability that all of these four independent events will occur is 1/30 × 1/2 × 1/30 × 1/2 or 1/3600. The mother who has one affected child has a risk of being a carrier that is equal to 1. The probability that her child will have Tay-Sachs disease is, therefore, 1 × 1/2 × 1/30 × 1/2 or 1/120. The joint probability of the mother who is an Ashkenazi Jew and the father who is not is 1/30 × 1/2 × 1/300 × 1/2 or 1/36,000.

279–281. The answers are: 279-D, 280-E, 281-B. *(Gelehrter, pp 49–68. Thompson, 5/e, pp 143–166.)* According to the Hardy-Weinberg equilibrium the frequency of heterozygotes $(2pq)$ is twice the square root of the rare homozygote frequency (q^2). The man whose brother has cystic fibrosis has a 2/3 chance of being a carrier and a 1/20 chance that his wife is a carrier. His risk for an affected child is 2/3 × 1/20 × 1/4 = 1/120. The African-American man and woman each have a 1/8 chance of having sickle trait with a 1/64 × 1/4 = 1/256 chance of having a child with sickle cell anemia. The grandmother with cystic fibrosis mandates that her children are carriers, so that each cousin has a 1/2 chance of being a carrier with a 1/2 × 1/2 × 1/4 = 1/16 chance of having an affected child, thus illustrating the effects of consanguinity.

282–284. The answers are: 282-D, 283-B, 284-E. *(Gelehrter, pp 49–65. Thompson, 5/e, pp 143–165.)* For a given individual, parents, siblings, and children represent first-degree relatives; grandparents, aunts, uncles, nephews, nieces, and half-siblings represent second-degree relatives, and first cousins represent third-degree relatives. Similar degrees of relationships indicate similar risks for common birth defects that follow polygenic inheritance as indicated in the question. In actuality, the risks are somewhat different for various types of common birth defects and may increase or decrease greatly according to the sex of the individual at risk.

285–287. The answers are: 285-A, 286-C, 287-E. *(Gelehrter, pp 49–65. Thompson, 5/e, pp 143–165.)* Allele frequencies indicate the likelihood for that allele to occur at a locus. The proportion of individuals with a given blood type are represented by the number of genotypes that yield the blood type multiplied by their likelihood to occur. For example, type B results from genotypes BO, OB, and BB; the probability that alleles B and O will occur together is $0.1 \times 0.7 = 0.07$ and that homozygous B will occur is $0.1 \times 0.1 = 0.01$. Type B individuals will constitute $70 + 70 + 10 = 150$ individuals per 1000. Since the ABO and MN blood group loci are not linked, their allele frequencies will be independent of one another. The proportion of type B, N individuals will be the joint probability that type B individuals (0.15) will be homozygous for allele N—that is, $0.16 = 0.15 \times 0.16 = 0.240 = 24$ per 1000.

Clinical Genetics

DIRECTIONS: Each question below contains five suggested responses. Select the **one best** response to each question.

288. Which of the following statements regarding most human cancers is true?

(A) They are nongenetic
(B) They are inherited in an autosomal dominant fashion
(C) They are inherited in an autosomal recessive fashion
(D) They follow a multifactorial model
(E) They are caused by germ-line mutations

289. The empiric risk of birth defects in first-cousin matings is

(A) equal to the baseline risk in all pregnancies
(B) 2 to 3 times the normal baseline risk
(C) 10 times the normal baseline risk
(D) 100 times the normal baseline risk

290. Screening of newborns for phenylketonuria (PKU) generally uses the Guthrie test. For each 100 positive Guthrie tests, how many infants will have classic PKU (phenylalanine > 20 mg/dL)?

(A) 100
(B) 50
(C) 25
(D) 10
(E) 5

DIRECTIONS: Each numbered question or incomplete statement below is NEGATIVELY phrased. Select the **one best** lettered response.

291. Newborn screening is available for several metabolic disorders, including phenylketonuria (PKU), maple syrup urine disease (MSUD), and biotinidase deficiency. Important factors to consider before initiating a newborn screening program include all the following EXCEPT the

(A) severity of the disorder
(B) community acceptance
(C) cost
(D) benefit of early detection
(E) availability of prenatal diagnosis for the disorder

292. Initial tests that may help to diagnose an inborn error of metabolism include all the following EXCEPT

(A) electrolytes
(B) complete blood count (CBC)
(C) karyotype
(D) plasma amino acids
(E) blood gas

293. Metabolic disease may include all the following signs and symptoms EXCEPT

(A) metabolic acidosis
(B) respiratory alkalosis
(C) metabolic alkalosis
(D) unusual odors
(E) seizures

294. Facial dysmorphisms may be seen in all the following conditions EXCEPT

(A) chromosomal abnormalities
(B) multifactorial conditions
(C) autosomal dominant conditions
(D) metabolic disease
(E) sepsis

295. Factors known to affect teratogenicity include all the following EXCEPT

(A) maternal genotype
(B) paternal exposure
(C) fetal genotype
(D) dosage of agent
(E) timing of exposure to agent

296. Which of the following conditions is NOT inherited in an autosomal dominant fashion?

(A) Neurofibromatosis
(B) Phenylketonuria
(C) Adult polycystic kidney disease
(D) Huntington's disease
(E) Marfan syndrome

297. All the following traits are X-linked EXCEPT

(A) sickle cell disease
(B) hemophilia A
(C) Duchenne's muscular dystrophy
(D) glucose-6-phosphate dehydrogenase deficiency
(E) color-blindness

298. Indications for genetic counseling include all the following EXCEPT

(A) consanguinity
(B) family history of cystic fibrosis
(C) family history of congenital infection
(D) teratogen exposure
(E) advanced maternal age

299. Data that support the conclusion that human tumors are generally monoclonal include all the following EXCEPT

(A) immunoglobulin rearrangements are consistent within tumors
(B) tumor cells express the same X-linked alleles
(C) translocations are present in all cells of a given tumor
(D) translocations activate a growth-promoting gene
(E) Southern blots of tumor cells demonstrate single bands when evaluating specific rearranged DNA segments

300. All the following statements regarding specific oncogenes are true EXCEPT

(A) less than 20 have been described
(B) they resemble transforming retroviruses
(C) they encode receptor genes
(D) they are involved in signal transmission between receptors and the nucleus
(E) they may regulate DNA transcription

301. Proto-oncogenes may be activated by all the following mechanisms EXCEPT

(A) single-point mutations
(B) chromsomal translocations
(C) loss of tumor suppressor genes
(D) amplification
(E) truncation

DIRECTIONS: Each group of questions below consists of lettered headings followed by a set of numbered items. For each numbered item select the **one** lettered heading with which it is **most** closely associated. Each lettered heading may be used **once, more than once or not at all.**

Questions 302–304

Match each of the following clinical situations with the term that best describes it.

(A) Sequence
(B) Syndrome
(C) Disruption
(D) Deformation
(E) Single malformation

302. Mandibular hypoplasia in utero leads to a posteriorly located tongue, which leads to restriction or closure of palatal shelves, resulting in cleft palate

303. An infant with trisomy 13 who has holoprosencephaly, defects of the eye, nose, cleft lip and palate, polydactyly, and scalp defects

304. A mother and child with cleft palate, unusual facies, including a flat face, a depressed nasal bridge, and myopia

Questions 305–307

Match each of the following descriptions with the term that best describes it.

(A) Sequence
(B) Syndrome
(C) Disruption
(D) Deformation
(E) Malformation

305. Crowding because of uterine fibroid tumor or oligohydramnios (abnormality extrinsic to structure)

306. Decreased perfusion because of vascular blow-out (abnormality extrinsic to structure)

307. Horseshoe kidney (abnormality intrinsic to structure)

Questions 308–310

Match each of the following statements with the type of counseling they exemplify.

(A) Nondirective genetic counseling
(B) Preconceptional counseling
(C) Prenatal counseling
(D) Informative counseling
(E) Supportive counseling

308. An infant has multiple congenital anomalies that require an extensive evaluation to establish a diagnosis

309. A first-born son has cystic fibrosis, which implies a 2/3 chance that his sister is a carrier

310. The high risk for birth defects in pregnancies with uncontrolled diabetes means that women must establish good management of their disease when deciding to attempt a pregnancy

Questions 311–312

A couple has a child who has been diagnosed with medium-chain acyl–coenzyme A (CoA) dehydrogenase deficiency (MCAD), an autosomal recessive condition that affects the body's ability to metabolize medium-chain fatty acids. This couple is now expecting another child. Match the following pregnancy outcomes with the probability of occurrence.

(A) 2/3
(B) 1/2
(C) 1/3
(D) 1/4

311. Affected child

312. Carrier of the gene for MCAD

Questions 313–315

The metabolite that accumulates in alkaptonuria and is responsible for dark urine is homogentisic acid (HA). The pathway for HA synthesis begins with dietary phenylalanine (PA) that is converted successively by enzymes E1 through E4 to tyrosine (Y), p-hydroxyphenylpyruvate (PHP), HA, and maleylacetoacetic acid (MA).

diet→PA→Y→PHP→HA→MA
intestine E1 E2   E3   E4

Match the statements about this pathway listed below with their likely consequences.

(A) No effect because of enzyme reserve
(B) Accumulation of all intermediates, depending on regulation
(C) Deficiency of all intermediates, depending on regulation
(D) Accumulation of HA, deficiency of MA
(E) Accumulation of PA, deficiency of Y

313. Deficiency of enzyme E4 as in alkaptonuria

314. Fifty percent activity of enzyme E4 in most tissues

315. Dietary restriction of PA

Questions 316–318

Some genetic disorders are more prevalent in certain ethnic groups. Match each of the following diseases with the ethnic group most likely to be affected by it.

(A) Ashkenazi Jews
(B) African Americans
(C) Northern Europeans
(D) Greeks
(E) Scandinavians

316. Alpha-thalassemia

317. Tay-Sachs disease

318. Cystic fibrosis

Questions 319–321

Match the following situations with the appropriate genetic principle.

(A) Pleiotropy
(B) Allelic heterogeneity
(C) Locus heterogeneity
(D) Linkage disequilibrium
(E) Variable expressivity

319. Bleeding associated with both factor VIII and factor IX deficiencies

320. Ornithine transcarbamylase deficiency (OTCD) caused by both single, base-pair deletions and substitutions

321. Tall, thin body habitus and lens dislocation seen in both homocystinuria and Marfan syndrome

Questions 322–324

A patient with the Marfan syndrome is evaluated at a clinic. He is noted to have a tall, thin body habitus, loose joints, and arachnodactyly (spider fingers) that allows the maneuver shown in the top figure below. Ophthalmologic examination reveals lens dislocation shown in the bottom figure below. An echocardiogram reveals dilatation of the aortic root. A family history reveals that his parents are medically normal, but that his paternal grandfather and great-grandfather died in their forties with lens dislocation and dissecting aortic aneurysms. A sister is found to have a similar body habitus, dilatation of the aortic root, and normal lenses. Match each of the following features of this case with the corresponding genetic principles.

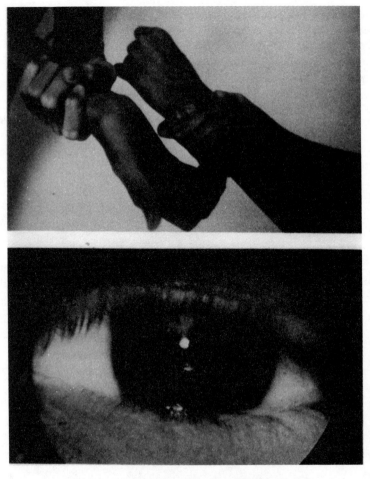

(See next page for choices and questions.)

(A) Pleiotropy
(B) Founder effect
(C) Variable expressivity
(D) Incomplete penetrance
(E) Genetic heterogeneity

322. There is involvement of the skeletal, ophthalmologic, and cardiac systems

323. The parents are unaffected, but the grandfather and great-grandfather are affected

324. The sister does not have lens dislocation

Questions 325–327

Match each clinical situation listed below with the most appropriate explanation for it.

(A) Alteration in regulatory control
(B) DNA tumor virus
(C) Most common genetic alteration in human cancer
(D) Seen in patients with Down syndrome
(E) Two-hit hypothesis of Knudson

325. In Burkitt's lymphoma, a reciprocal translocation introduces a proto-oncogene into the immunoglobulin heavy-chain locus

326. In retinoblastoma, there is a loss of the allele on both chromosomes

327. The presence of the Philadelphia chromosome

Questions 328–330

A 2-year-old child presents with the complaint that her urine turned black on the bedsheets after an episode of bed-wetting. The parents are aware of no dietary changes, and the family history is negative except for the fact that the parents are first cousins. The physician collects a urine sample from the child and from a parent; the child's urine turns relatively dark (*left* in the figure below) after incubation at room temperature. Assuming that this is a genetic disease with an abnormal allele (a) frequency of 1/100, match each of the following individuals with the probable risks of transmitting this disease.

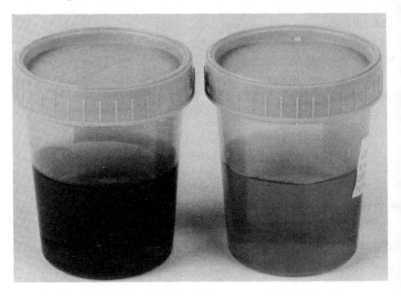

    (A) 1/4
    (B) 1/8
    (C) 1/12
    (D) 1/100
    (E) 1/300

328. Risk of proband to transmit the disease if she marries her uncle

329. Risk of unaffected sibling of proband to transmit the disease with an unrelated spouse

330. Risk of unaffected sibling of proband to transmit the disease if she marries her uncle

Questions 331–333

The proband from the pedigree shown in the figure below consults the physician about her family history of a bleeding disorder. She has medical records that document a diagnosis of von Willebrand's disease (vWD) in her affected father and uncle. The most common mode of inheritance of vWD is autosomal dominant. Based on the probable conclusions of the physician about the mode of inheritance, match each individual listed below with his or her probable risk.

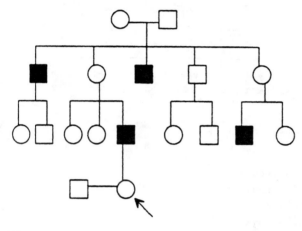

(A) 100 percent
(B) 75 percent
(C) 50 percent
(D) 25 percent
(E) 11 percent

331. The proband's risk to have an affected child

332. The proband's risk to have an affected child if she married her affected uncle

333. The risk that the proband's aunt is a carrier given that she has three unaffected boys

Questions 334–336

The pedigree below shows individuals affected with autosomal recessive xeroderma pigmentosum. Match each individual listed below with his or her risk to be a carrier (heterozygote).

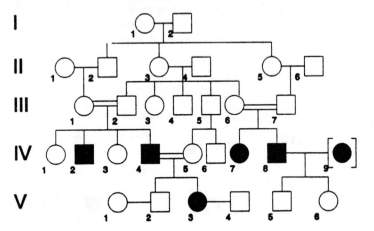

(A) 100 percent
(B) 75 percent
(C) 67 percent
(D) 50 percent
(E) 33 percent

334. II-2

335. III-5

336. V-5

Clinical Genetics

Answers

288. The answer is D. *(Gelehrter, pp 229–252. Thompson, 5/e, pp 365–381.)* Although certain cancer syndromes are inherited in a Mendelian fashion, most human cancers cannot be explained using simple patterns of single-gene inheritance. Nevertheless, genetics does play an important role in the inheritance and development of cancer. Although more complicated than most multifactorial disorders, human cancers generally follow a multifactorial model. The greater the number and closer the relationship of relatives with cancer, the greater the risk. Additionally, more severe disease may result in an increased risk of disease in relatives. Certainly, environmental influences are important in the development of cancer (e.g., the relationship between cigarette smoking and lung cancer).

289. The answer is B. *(Gelehrter, pp 395–410. Thompson, 5/e, pp 69–70, 262–269.)* It is generally believed that all people are heterozygous for at least several genes for rare recessive disorders. Consanguinity increases the chance that a child will inherit two genes that are identical by descent. Empirically, the increased risk for the child of a first-cousin mating to have a serious birth defect or genetic disease is approximately two to three times the baseline risk (i.e., 5 to 6 percent).

290. The answer is E. *(Gelehrter, pp 270–275. Thompson, 5/e, pp 407–409.)* Newborn screening for phenylketonuria (PKU) is provided in the United States and in most other developed nations. The screening method most commonly employed is the Guthrie test. Drops of blood from an infant are placed on bits of filter paper. Disks soaked with blood are placed on agar plates that contain thienylalanine and that are growing *Bacillus subtilis*. The thienylalanine inhibits the growth of the bacteria; however, when phenylalanine is present in sufficient amounts in the blood, this inhibition is overcome and the bacteria continue to grow. Standardized disks are used to set a positive result at over 4 mg/dL of phenylalanine. Although classic PKU presents with phenylalanine levels greater than 20 mg/dL, levels are set low to avoid problems with false-negative results. Additionally, setting test limits at this level allows for the detection of other PKU variants, which may present with lower levels of phenylalanine.

291. The answer is E. *(Gelehrter, pp 270–275. Thompson, 5/e, pp 407–409.)* Screening programs for newborns are currently in place in all 50 states. Beginning in the 1960s, these programs were established to identify infants with treatable genetic diseases. In deciding whether to establish a screening program and for which diseases to screen, many issues must be addressed. The frequency and severity of the disorders must be established. In general, disorders included in screening programs should have an efficacious method of treatment, which, if instituted early, will prevent serious consequences of the disorder. The test used to detect the disorder should be reliable, accurate, safe, and relatively inexpensive so that the cost of the screening is outweighed by the savings of early treatment and prevention of serious sequelae. There must be resources to assure effective treatment and follow-up once affected individuals are identified. The availability of prenatal testing is not a prerequisite for a successful newborn screening program.

292. The answer is C. *(Scriver, 6/e, pp 3–53.)* Primary care physicians are taking a major role in the diagnosis and treatment of genetic diseases. If the primary care physician does not recognize the signs and symptoms of metabolic disease, a diagnosis will not be made, treatment will not be initiated, and families will be unaware of their risks in future pregnancies. Several simple and relatively inexpensive tests allow for the diagnosis of most inborn errors of metabolism. These tests include a complete blood count (CBC), electrolytes, blood gas, plasma ammonia, amino acids, and urine organic acids. The karyotype is generally normal in individuals with metabolic disease.

293. The answer is C. *(Scriver, 6/e, pp 3–53.)* Several simple tests greatly aid in the diagnosis of metabolic disease. First, it is important to remember that infants with inborn errors of metabolism may present in very nonspecific ways, such as with lethargy, vomiting, seizures, coma, and death. It is important to note if there are any unusual odors to the infant's urine or skin. Elevated levels of organic acids cause a metabolic acidosis. Ammonia is a primary respiratory stimulant and elevated levels cause a respiratory alkalosis. An increased anion gap is also an important clue to the diagnosis of metabolic disease. Metabolic alkalosis is not a common feature of metabolic disease.

294. The answer is E. *(Scriver, 6/e, pp 3–53.)* Facial dysmorphisms are common features of various syndromes that are caused by chromosomal abnormalities. They are also frequently seen in persons with autosomal dominant and autosomal recessive syndromes. Multifactorial conditions, such as cleft lip and palate, also give a dysmorphic appearance to the face. Certain rare inborn errors of metabolism, such as glutaricacidemia, type II, and the Zellweger syndrome, a disorder of peroxisomal metabolism, also are associated with facial dysmorphisms. Acquired disorders, such as sepsis, are not associated with dysmorphic facies.

295. The answer is B. *(Thompson, 5/e, pp 392–394.)* A teratogen is an agent that causes a malformation or raises the incidence of malformations. The dosage of teratogen to which a fetus is exposed affects the response to that agent. The mother's ability to metabolize the agent, a factor related to her genotype, also plays a role. The genotype of the mother is also important in situations in which the mother has a genetic defect, such as phenylketonuria (PKU). In maternal PKU, the elevated levels of phenylalanine are teratogenic to the fetus. Fetal genotype also affects response to a teratogen. The effects of a given teratogen may be different, depending on the stage of development at which the fetus is exposed. Despite publicity about "agent orange," paternal exposure is unlikely to affect the teratogenicity of a given agent.

296. The answer is B. *(Gelehrter, pp 59–88. Isselbacher, 13/e, pp 342–350. Thompson, 5/e, pp 29–36.)* Although it would be impossible to remember the pattern of inheritance for all genetic disorders, certain conditions are either relatively common or represent classic examples of genetic disease. All the disorders listed in the question are inherited in an autosomal dominant fashion with the exception of phenylketonuria (PKU), which is an autosomal recessive inborn error of metabolism.

297. The answer is A. *(Gelehrter, pp 59–88. Isselbacher, 13/e, pp 342–350. Thompson, 5/e, pp 29–36.)* X-linked recessive traits, such as hemophilia A, Duchenne's muscular dystrophy, glucose-6-phosphate dehydrogenase deficiency, and color-blindness, are inherited in an oblique fashion. They are much commoner in men than women. Sickle cell anemia is an autosomal recessive hemoglobinopathy, which is relatively common in African Americans.

298. The answer is C. *(Gelehrter, pp 262–270. Thompson, 5/e, pp 395–409.)* There are many indications for genetic counseling. These include advanced maternal age, family history of birth defects or other known or suspected genetic disease, unexplained mental retardation, and consanguinity. Although not technically a genetic problem, teratogen exposure is also generally accepted as an indication for genetic counseling. Although a history of congenital infection requires that medical information be given to the family, this is not a heritable disorder and, therefore, is not an indication for genetic counseling. However, should a pregnant woman herself contract an infection, such as rubella, which may be teratogenic, genetic counseling should be offered.

299. The answer is D. *(Gelehrter, pp 229–252. Thompson, 5/e, pp 365–381.)* In most cases, tumors arise from a single ancestral cell that has undergone some mutational event (somatic mutation). Studies to support this contention have shown that all cells within that tumor have identical DNA makeups. The original evidence for this was the finding that all cells in a tumor from a woman who was heterozygous for a mutation at the glucose-6-phosphate dehydrogenase (G6PD) locus expressed the same allele. Since X-inactivation is a random event, it would be expected that the normal allele would be expressed in some cells and the mutant allele in others, unless all cells had derived from a single cell. Other supporting evidence includes the fact that, when a translocation is present, it is seen in all cells of the tumor and none of the normal cells. additionally, the same immunoglobulin or other gene rearrangements have been seen in all tumor cells. These rearrangements can be demonstrated on Southern blots, using DNA from tumor cells and comparing it to DNA from normal tissue.

300. The answer is A. *(Gelehrter, pp 229–252. Thompson, 5/e, pp 365–381.)* Proto-oncogenes are genes that perform important normal functions involved in the regulation of cell growth. Unfortunately, when these genes are mutated or overexpressed, they may result in malignant transformation. The mutated form of the gene is generally referred to as an oncogene. More than 50 human oncogenes have been described. Some oncogenes are identical to genes for both growth factors and growth-factor receptors. Other oncogenes act in the signal transmission pathway from receptor to the nucleus. Others are involved in the regulation of transcription or DNA replication. Many oncogenes resemble RNA retroviruses, which use reverse transcriptase to make a DNA copy of their sequence. The DNA from these viruses, in turn, integrates itself into chromosomal DNA from a host and induces malignant transformation.

301. The answer is C. *(Gelehrter, pp 229–252. Thompson, 5/e, pp 365–381.)* Proto-oncogenes may be mutated in multiple ways to create oncogenes. Single-point mutations may lead to the synthesis of an abnormal gene product. Chromsomal translocations may juxtapose genes in such a way as to allow for overexpression. For example, in Burkitt's lymphoma, a translocation places the myc locus near the heavy-chain immunoglobulin gene. This appears to deregulate the oncogene and allow it to be greatly overexpressed, resulting in lymphomatous transformation. Amplification of an oncogene also allows for overexpression. Truncation of a cell surface receptor has been noted. This appears to result in a gene that behaves as if it were continually being stimulated and, thus, grows in an unrestrained fashion. In contrast to oncogenes that promote abnormal cell growth, tumor suppressor genes block abnormal growth. It is only when these genes are lost that malignant transformation occurs.

302–304. The answers are: 302-A, 303-B, 304-B. *(Thompson, 5/e, pp 391–393.)* A sequence such as the Pierre-Robin sequence described in the question is a pattern of anomalies that originates from a single prior defect or mechanical factor. A syndrome is a pattern of multiple malformations or anomalies thought to be pathogenetically related but embryologically unrelated. Syndromes may be caused by chromosomal abnormalities as in the case of trisomy 13, or they may also be Mendelian disorders as in the case of the mother and child who have the Stickler syndrome, an autosomal dominant defect in collagen.

305–307. The answers are: 305-D, 306-C, 307-E. *(Thompson, 5/e, pp 391–393.)* Anomalous development of an organ primordium may be due to intrinsic factors or to extrinsic interference. Early and intrinsic abnormalities are termed *malformations,* and these point to Mendelian, chromosomal, or polygenic causes. *Disruptions* and *deformations* often reflect the operation of mechanical factors that are less likely to be genetic. If a single abnormality produces a chain of embryologically related events—as with early urethral obstruction that leads to abdominal distention, resulting in abdominal muscle wall weakness and excess skin (prune belly)—then the pattern of anomalies is called a *sequence.* If a single abnormality produces a pattern of defects that seem embryologically unrelated, this is called a *syndrome* (literally, *running together*). Syndromes have a high chance of having a Mendelian or chromosomal cause, while sequences imply the polygenic or sporadic inheritance of single birth defects.

308–310. The answers are: 308-D, 309-A, 310-B. *(Gelehrter, pp 255–286.)* Genetic counseling is usually nondirective; that is, it provides facts without bias as to the patient's reproductive decisions. *Preconceptual counseling* is an important goal for all genetic or teratogenic diseases so that appropriate risks and management are known before the pregnancy is initiated. *Prenatal counseling* involves couples who wish to become pregnant or expectant couples who seek advice on risks, prenatal diagnostic options, and perinatal management. *Supportive counseling* is within the expertise of every physician and involves acknowledging a disease with genetic implications and providing a plan for evaluation and diagnosis. Since many genetic events are crises—for example, the birth of an abnormal child—there is a natural overlap of the family's inability to hear detailed counseling information and the physician's inability to provide it until tests or consultations are obtained. *Informative counseling* provides the details of disease and recurrence risks to concerned family members. It requires a precise diagnosis or diagnostic category.

311–312. The answers are: 311-D, 312-B. *(Gelehrter, pp 36–39. Thompson, 5/e, pp 66–72.)* Assuming that nonpaternity or an unusual method of inheritance is not operative, the parents of a child with an autosomal recessive condition are obligate heterozygotes. Therefore, their risk of having a child with medium-chain acyl–coenzyme A (CoA) dehydrogenase deficiency (MCAD) is 1/4 or 25 percent for each future pregnancy. Prior to delivery, when the clinical status of the child is unknown, the risk that the child will be heterozygous for a mutation at the MCAD locus is 1/2 or 50 percent.

313–315. The answers are: 313-D, 314-A, 315-C. *(Gelehrter, p 125–158. Thompson, 5/e, pp 271–316.)* Inherited disorders of metabolism usually result from severe enzyme deficiencies (0 to 5 percent residual activity) with consequent elevation or depletion of metabolites. Some elevated metabolites, such as phenylalanine, are probably toxic to the brain and cause mental retardation, while others, like homogentisic acid, are deposited in cartilage and cause arthritis. Metabolite deficiency is exemplified by the lack of purines needed for immune response in adenosine deaminase deficiency. Therapy for metabolic disorders is based on removing the accumulating substance, supplementing substrate deficiencies, or both. Because enzymes are present in amounts greater than needed for usual pathway demands (enzyme reserve), reduction to 50 percent levels usually has no effect. This is the usual reason that heterozygotes (carriers) for autosomal recessive diseases are normal.

316–318. The answers are: 316-B, 317-A, 318-C. *(Isselbacher, 13/e, p 342.)* One important aspect of taking a family history is to determine the ethnic origin of the family. Many genetic disorders have an increased frequency in specific ethnic groups. African Americans have an increased frequency of many hemoglobinopathies including Hb S, Hb C, persistent Hb F, and α- and β-thalassemias. Greeks and other Mediterranean peoples have an increased frequency of β-thalassemia. Ashkenazi Jews have an increased risk for many disorders, including Tay-Sachs disease, the adult form of Gaucher's disease, familial dysautonomia, and Bloom syndrome. Northern Europeans have an increased risk for cystic fibrosis, and Scandinavians have an increased incidence of α_1-antitrypsin deficiency.

319–321. The answers are: 319-C, 320-B, 321-C. *(Gelehrter, pp 29–36. Thompson, 5/e, p 57.)* Genetic heterogeneity refers to the fact that different mutations may cause similar phenotypes. This may be further divided into allelic and nonallelic (locus) heterogeneity. Allelic heterogeneity implies that there are different mutations at the same locus, which both result in similar disease. In locus heterogeneity, mutations occur at different loci, yet the phenotype is similar. Locus heterogeneity also explains why certain disorders may be inherited in several different fashions. It is especially important to recognize the possibility of genetic heterogeneity when counseling patients in regard to recurrence risks.

322–324. The answers are: 322-A, 323-D, 324-C. *(Gelehrter, pp 29–36. Thompson, 5/e, pp 59–66, 83–90.)* Although a mutation at a single locus generally alters a single gene, the result being the abnormal synthesis or lack of production of a single RNA molecule or polypeptide chain, the results of this mutation may be far-reaching. When there are multiple phenotypic effects involving multiple systems, it is referred to as pleiotropy. Penetrance is the all or none expression of an abnormal genotype, whereas expressivity is the degree of expression of that genotype. Incomplete or reduced penetrance implies that some individuals have a mutant allele with absolutely no phenotypic expression of that allele. Variable expressivity implies that all individuals with a mutant allele have some phenotypic effects, although the severity and range of effects differ in different people.

325–327. The answers are: 325-A, 326-E, 327-D. *(Gelehrter, pp 365–381. Thompson, 5/e, pp 229–252.)* In Burkitt's lymphoma, a B-cell lymphoma that usually occurs in childhood, chromosomal translocations are frequently noted. The most common of these rearrangements is the reciprocal translocation of chromosomes 8 and 14. The result of this is to place the c-myc proto-oncogene from 8q24 into the immunoglobulin heavy-chain locus at 14q32. Since immunoglobulin genes are actively transcribed, this move alters the normal regulatory control of c-myc.

Retinoblastoma is a tumor of retinal cells that occurs in young children. It can be seen in both sporadic and familial forms. Familial cases appear to be inherited as an autosomal dominant trait with incomplete penetrance. In familial cases, tumors tend to involve both eyes, and there may be multiple lesions in each eye. This has led to the two-hit hypothesis originally developed by Knudson. Because the condition is inherited, one mutation must have a germ-line origin. However, a second somatic mutational event is required to begin malignant transformation. In sporadic cases, two somatic mutational events must take place. Since these somatic mutations are relatively rare events, it is extremely unlikely for more than one tumor to develop. It is curious that, although retinoblastoma is inherited in a dominant fashion, tumor development is a recessive event, requiring the inactivation of both alleles. Mutation or loss of the p53 gene is the most common genetic alteration found in human cancer.

The Philadelphia chromosome is the name given to the translocation t(9:22)(q34:q11). This translocation is seen in almost all patients with chronic myelogenous leukemia (CML) and in a percentage of patients with acute lymphoblastic leukemia (ALL). The Philadelphia chromosome is seen with increased frequency in individuals with Down syndrome.

328–330. The answers are: 328-A, 329-E, 330-C. *(Thompson, 5/e, pp 53–72.)* The history of the 2-year-old girl suggests alkaptonuria (black urine), which was one of the first genetic disorders to be recognized as Mendelian by Sir Archibald Garrod. Consanguinity of the parents always suggests autosomal recessive disorders, as does the metabolic abnormality implied by urine with an unusual color or odor. The parents must both be genotypes Aa with a 1/4 risk for another aa child. The proband must be genotype aa, and her prospective unrelated spouse has a 2*pq* and, thus, a 2 × 1/100 = 1/50 chance to be an Aa carrier, which results in a 1 × 1/50 × 1/2 = 1/100 chance of having an affected aa child. If she marries her uncle, then he has a 1/2 chance to be genotype Aa with a 1 × 1/2 × 1/2 = 1/4 chance of having an affected child. The unaffected sibling will have a 2/3 chance to be Aa with a 2/3 × 1/50 × 1/4 = 1/300 chance of having an affected child if her spouse is unrelated and a 2/3 × 1/2 × 1/4 = 1/12 chance if she marries her uncle.

331–333. The answers are: 331-D, 332-C, 333-E. *(Gelehrter, pp 27–47. Thompson, 5/e, pp 53–73.)* The pedigree that accompanies the question is much more suggestive of X-linked recessive than autosomal dominant inheritance because of its oblique pattern and predominance of affected males. Reference to Dr. Victor McKusick's *Mendelian Inheritance in Man* reveals a rare X-linked recessive form of von Willebrand's disease that supports this conclusion. The proband is an obligate carrier since her father is affected, and she has a 1/2 chance of transmitting the abnormal allele and a 1/2 chance of having a son. Her risk of having an affected child is thus 1/2 × 1/2 = 1/4. Her uncle would also have an abnormal allele on his X chromosome, which results in the risk of 1/2 for an affected male and 1/2 for an affected female with abnormal alleles on both X chromosomes. Three unaffected boys changes the aunt's risk from 1/2 chance of being a carrier to 1/9 (11 percent), using Bayesian counseling.

334–336. The answers are: 334-A, 335-A, 336-A. *(Gelehrter, pp 27–47. Thompson, 5/e, pp 53–72.)* Xeroderma pigmentosum (XP) is an autosomal recessive disorder in which defective DNA repair causes sensitivity to sunlight, skin lesions, and cancer. Autosomal recessive inheritance is supported by the consanguinity in the pedigree. The spouse (IV-9) of individual IV-8 has severe disease and is likely to be unrelated although she is an adoptee. If she had the same recessive disease, both parents would be homozygous abnormal, and all their children would be affected. The most likely explanation is genetic heterogeneity with the parents' having mutations at different loci that produce similar clinical symptoms. The presence of up to five different loci responsible for XP is suggested by coculture of fibroblasts from different patients and noting whether they can restore each other's repair defects (*complementation*). If different loci are involved, then the offspring would be carriers for both abnormal alleles but would not be affected.

For IV-2 to have been affected (homozygous abnormal), II-2 must have transmitted the abnormal allele to III-1 and, thus, must be a carrier. The same is true for III-5 in order for V-3 to be affected. V-5 must be a carrier because a parent is homozygous affected. IV-1 is an unaffected sibling of IV-2 and cannot be homozygous abnormal. Given the abnormal allele x and the normal allele X, her remaining alternatives for genotypes are Xx (x from the mother), xX (x from the father), or XX—giving her a 2/3 chance of being a carrier.

Reproductive Genetics

DIRECTIONS: Each question below contains five suggested responses. Select the **one best** response to each question.

337. Every prenatal evaluation should include which of the following diagnostic procedures?

(A) Level I ultrasound
(B) Chorionic villus sampling (CVS)
(C) Doppler analysis
(D) Amniocentesis
(E) Genetic counseling

338. What is the frequency of pregnancy termination after prenatal diagnosis?

(A) > 90 percent
(B) 50 percent
(C) 25 percent
(D) 10 percent
(E) < 5 percent

339. A woman undergoes chorionic villus sampling (CVS), and a fetal karyotype of 46,XX/47,XX,+16 is found. The patient decides to continue the pregnancy, hoping that the abnormal cell line was an artifact. Subsequent fetal growth was delayed, but a karyotype on the small-for-gestational-age infant was 46,XX. These findings are best explained by a

(A) true mosaicism in the embryo with later predominance of the normal cell line
(B) mosaicism as an artifact of cell culture
(C) confined placental mosaicism with trisomy 16 in the fetus
(D) true mosaicism in the early embryo with correction to uniparental disomy 16 in the fetus
(E) trisomy 16 in the newborn infant

DIRECTIONS: Each numbered question or incomplete statement below is NEGATIVELY phrased. Select the **one best** lettered response.

340. Amniocentesis is indicated for all the following situations EXCEPT

(A) prior child with mental retardation
(B) maternal age >35
(C) prior child with spina bifida
(D) prior child with inborn error of metabolism
(E) prior child with chromosomal abnormality

341. Genetic counseling helps a couple do all the following EXCEPT

(A) understand the medical facts
(B) understand the mode of inheritance and recurrence risks
(C) adjust to the condition
(D) rule out the need for prenatal diagnosis when pregnancy termination is an unacceptable alternative
(E) select a course of action

342. Neural tube defects, such as spina bifida or anencephaly, can be diagnosed by all of the following prenatal procedures EXCEPT

(A) ultrasound at 16 weeks' gestation
(B) maternal serum α-fetoprotein (MSAFP) levels
(C) amniotic fluid α-fetoprotein (AFP) levels
(D) amniotic fluid acetylcholinesterase levels
(E) fetal karyotyping

343. Biochemical prenatal diagnosis of inborn errors of metabolism requires all the following EXCEPT

(A) a biochemical assay that can be used on cell culture or amniotic fluid
(B) a biochemical defect that is expressed in amniotic fluid, amniocytes, or chorionic villi
(C) an assay that separates individuals with 50 percent enzyme levels from those with 0 to 10 percent levels
(D) the defect to be autosomal recessive
(E) results to be available within 2 to 4 weeks

344. Prenatal diagnosis provides all the following functions EXCEPT

(A) it provides reassurance that the fetus is not affected with a specific disease
(B) it allows couples to make an informed decision as to whether to continue the pregnancy
(C) it lowers the incidence of many diseases by allowing prenatal detection and termination of affected fetuses
(D) it provides screening strategies for women over age 35 with higher risks for chromosomal disorders
(E) it indicates whether a fetus has a congenital heart defect

DIRECTIONS: Each group of questions below consists of lettered headings followed by a set of numbered items. For each numbered item select the **one** lettered heading with which it is **most** closely associated. Each lettered heading may be used **once, more than once or not at all.**

Questions 345–347

Match each of the procedures listed below with the characteristic that distinguishes it.

(A) 0.5 to 1 mL fetal blood
(B) 8 to 10 weeks' gestation
(C) 20 to 30 mL fluid volume
(D) All trimesters
(E) Maternal blood

345. Chorionic villus sampling (CVS)

346. Amniocentesis

347. Percutaneous umbilical blood sampling (PUBS)

Questions 348–350

Match the procedures listed below with the appropriate description.

(A) Results within 24 to 48 hours
(B) Results within 2 to 4 weeks
(C) Fetal blood flow
(D) Dating of pregnancy
(E) Fetal anomalies

348. Level I ultrasound

349. Level II ultrasound

350. Doppler analysis

Questions 351–353

A 33-year-old woman seeks genetic counseling for her first pregnancy. The couple's family and past medical histories were unremarkable. Measurement of maternal serum α-fetoprotein (MSAFP) concentration and level I ultrasound were performed at an estimated gestational age of 16 weeks. For each of the clinical situations listed below, select the appropriate diagnostic result.

(A) 20 ng/mL
(B) 5.5 multiples of means (MOM) for gestational age by ultrasound of 15½ weeks
(C) 1.0 MOM for gestational age by ultrasound of 15½ weeks
(D) 0.5 MOM for gestational age by ultrasound of 15½ weeks

351. Uninterpretable result

352. Possible fetal Down syndrome

353. Possible fetal death or twin pregnancy

Questions 354–356

A 37-year-old woman and her 45-year-old husband request genetic counseling regarding their second pregnancy. She undergoes amniocentesis and level I ultrasound study at an estimated 17 weeks' gestation. A single amniotic sample was obtained, and a photograph from the ultrasound is shown in the figure below. For each of the clinical situations listed below, select the appropriate result.

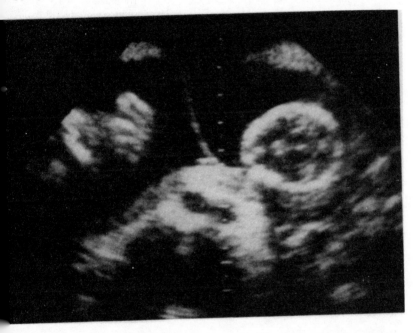

(A) Amniotic α-fetoprotein (AFP) concentration of 30 μg/mL; karyotype 46,XY
(B) Amniotic AFP 2 multiples of mean (MOM) for gestational age of 15 weeks estimated from ultrasound; karyotype 46,XY
(C) Amniotic AFP 6 MOM; karyotype 46,XY
(D) Amniotic AFP 2 MOM; karyotype 47,XY+21
(E) Amniotic AFP measures 30 μg/mL; karyotype 47,XY,+21

354. Normal twin gestation

355. Normal karyotype; AFP level uninterpretable unless correlated with population mean and gestational age

356. Possible spina bifida; normal karyotype in one twin

Questions 357–361

For each of the prenatal diagnostic methods listed below, select the clinical situation in which it would be appropriate.

(A) Couple whose child has cleft palate

(B) Couple whose child has trisomy 18; wants safest procedure

(C) Couple whose child has club foot

(D) Twin pregnancy

(E) Couple whose child has cerebral palsy

(F) Couple of British ancestry

(G) Couple whose child has Tay-Sachs disease and whose church and relatives strongly disapprove of prenatal diagnosis

(H) Threatened abortion

(I) Fetal anomalies detected by ultrasound at 16 weeks' gestation

357. Cordocentesis

358. Chorionic villus sampling (CVS)

359. Amniocentesis

360. Maternal serum α-fetoprotein (MSAFP)

361. No prenatal diagnosis available

Questions 362–364

For each of the diseases listed below, select the appropriate diagnostic method.

(A) Fetal DNA testing after parental mutations are determined

(B) Fetal karyotyping to determine sex

(C) Fetal karyotyping to determine chromosome number

(D) Hexosaminidase assay of chorionic villi

(E) Type II ultrasound and measurement of amniotic fluid α-fetoprotein (AFP)

362. Cystic fibrosis

363. Down syndrome

364. Nonspecific X-linked mental retardation

Questions 365–367

Match each of the following clinical procedures with the appropriate pregnancy risk.

- (A) 2 to 3 percent risk for fetal loss
- (B) 0.5 to 1 percent risk for fetal loss above spontaneous abortion rate
- (C) Same risk as B, plus ill-defined risk for limb defects
- (D) No known risk
- (E) Risk undetermined

365. Doppler analysis

366. Amniocentesis (15 to 17 weeks' gestation)

367. Prenatal diagnosis without follow-up counseling

Reproductive Genetics
Answers

337. The answer is E. *(Gelehrter, pp 275–283. Thompson, 5/e, pp 411–425.)* Genetic counseling is an essential component of every prenatal diagnostic test. Couples must understand their risks and options before selecting a prenatal diagnostic procedure. There must also be adequate provisions for explaining the results. Since additional obstetric procedures, such as pregnancy termination, may follow prenatal diagnosis, obstetricians need to be comprehensive and thorough with the genetic counseling process.

338. The answer is E. *(Gelehrter, pp 275–283. Thompson, 5/e, pp 411–425.)* Although autosomal and X-linked recessive disorders imply a 25 percent recurrence risk, most prenatal diagnostic procedures are performed because of advanced maternal age (> 35). With a risk ranging from about 1 to 2 percent at age 35 to a maximum of 5 percent at age 45, the overall frequency of elective pregnancy termination following prenatal diagnosis is only about 3 percent. Thus, 97 percent of couples are reassured by prenatal diagnostic procedures.

339. The answer is D. *(Gelehrter, pp 275–283. Thompson, 5/e, pp 411–425.)* Trisomy 16 in the fetus or newborn is ruled out by the normal karyotype, although undetected trisomy 16 mosaicism is possible. Confined placental mosaicism does occur, and trisomy 16 cells in the placenta could cause growth retardation in the normal fetus through placental insufficiency. Culture mosaicism is common with chorionic villus sampling (CVS), because normal maternal tissue (i.e., uterine decidua) is included with the villi. Because trisomy 16 is a severe anomaly, found in spontaneous abortions but not in live-births, mosaicism can easily arise through mitotic nondisjunction to produce normal cells. Since two number 16 chromosomes in the trisomic cell derive from one parent, there is a 1/3 chance that the other parental chromosome will be lost, resulting in uniparental disomy 16. Growth retardation is a common effect of uniparental disomy and has been specifically reported with uniparental disomy 16.

340. The answer is A. *(Gelehrter, pp 275–283. Thompson, 5/e, pp 411–425.)* Amniocentesis has a risk for inducing miscarriages of less than 0.5 percent; therefore, conditions with a recurrence risk of about 1 percent or higher are acceptable indications for the procedure. Mental retardation is not a specific diagnosis; thus, prenatal detection is not feasible. At age 35, the risk for Down syndrome plus other chromosomal anomalies approaches 1 percent. This figure also applies to any couple who already has a child with a chromosomal anomaly regardless of their age. Parents of a child with a neural tube defect (e.g., spina bifida or anencephaly) face a 2 percent recurrence risk. The usual autosomal recessive inheritance of metabolic disorders predicts a 25 percent risk after one affected child.

341. The answer is D. *(Gelehrter, pp 275–283. Thompson, 5/e, pp 411–425.)* Genetic counseling addresses the medical circumstances, inheritance and recurrence risks, impact of a given risk for a particular family, options for management, and adjustment to the circumstances of risk and disease. Genetic counseling is traditionally nondirective, which means that the counselor does not attempt to influence the family's decisions. While abortion is unacceptable to many couples, prenatal diagnosis may still be useful in guiding perinatal management and in preparing the couple.

342. The answer is E. *(Gelehrter, pp 275–283. Thompson, 5/e, pp 411–425.)* Any defect of the fetal skin may elevate the amniotic α-fetoprotein (AFP) level, causing a parallel rise of this substance in the maternal blood. Other causes of increased AFP include fetal kidney disease with leakage of fetal proteins into amniotic fluid. Mild forms of spina bifida or meningomyelocele may cover the skin so that the AFP is not elevated. Ultrasound is useful for these cases as it is possible to detect all but the very smallest defects. Acetylcholinesterase is an enzyme produced at high levels in neural tissue that is somewhat more specific than AFP for neural tube defects. Because neural tube defects are usually isolated birth defects in children with normal chromosomes, a fetal karyotype would not be helpful.

343. The answer is D. *(Gelehrter, pp 275–283. Thompson, 5/e, pp 411–425.)* Most inborn errors of metabolism have been explained by deficiencies of particular enzymes that can be assayed in skin fibroblasts. Such deficiencies have usually been found in the corresponding amniocytes or chorionic villi. Occasionally, the elevated substrate or deficient product of this enzyme reaction can be reliably assayed in body fluids, including amniotic fluid. Biochemical disorders such as Marfan syndrome are autosomal dominant and involve defects in connective tissue molecules. Because amniocyte or chorionic villus culture often requires 2 to 3 weeks, a reliable and rapid biochemical assay is needed for prenatal diagnosis. Most centers will not perform an abortion after 24 weeks' gestation.

344. The answer is C. *(Gelehrter, pp 275–283. Thompson, 5/e, pp 411–425.)* Many disorders detected by prenatal diagnosis are X-linked or autosomal recessive genetic diseases. For such diseases, most of the abnormal alleles are present in carriers rather than in affected individuals. This derives from the Hardy-Weinberg law where $2pq$ equals the carrier frequency and q^2 equals homozygote frequency. For the average disorder where q is 1/100 or less, 1/50 people will be carriers, while only 1/10,000 will be affected. Fetal echocardiography at 16 to 22 weeks' gestation will detect most fetal heart defects.

345–347. The answers are: 345-B, 346-C, 347-A. *(Gelehrter, pp 275–283. Thompson, 5/e, pp 411–425.)* Chorionic villus sampling (CVS) involves aspiration of placental trophoblast tissue at 8 to 10 weeks of pregnancy. Since trophoblast cells are of fetal origin, direct or culture analysis for chromosomes can document the fetal karyotype. Amniocentesis is routinely performed at 15 to 17 weeks of pregnancy and withdraws 20 to 30 mL of amniotic fluid and cells for fetal analysis. Early amniocentesis, which withdraws a smaller amount of fluid, may be performed at 12 to 14 weeks of pregnancy. Percutaneous umbilical blood sampling (PUBS) or cordocentesis is used to aspirate 0.5 to 1 mL of fetal blood from the umbilical vein after maternal transabdominal puncture.

348–350. The answers are: 348-D, 349-E, 350-C. *(Gelehrter, pp 275–283. Thompson, 5/e, pp 411–425.)* Level I ultrasound allows such general determinations as dating of pregnancy, determination of fetal and placental placement, and detection of twins. Level II ultrasound is more time-consuming and involves careful imaging of specific fetal organs for detection of anomalies. Doppler analysis uses continuous ultrasound waves to determine the direction and velocity of blood flow in the fetoplacental unit.

351–353. The answers are: 351-A, 352-D, 353-B. *(Gelehrter, pp 275–283. Thompson, 5/e, pp 411–425.)* Concentrations of maternal serum α-fetoprotein (MSAFP) are meaningful only if correlated with the population mean and gestational age. Alpha-fetoprotein (AFP) is a fetal homologue of albumin that rises early and decreases late in gestation. Leakage of fetal blood or amniotic fluid into the maternal bloodstream produces small but detectable amounts of AFP in maternal serum. The decreased rate of fetal growth and development seen with autosomal trisomies decreases MSAFP values, while leakage of AFP from open neural tube defects increases MSAFP values. Other fetal conditions that produce elevated amniotic fluid AFP and MSAFP values include twins, fetal death, and fetal anomalies that disrupt the skin or kidney (e.g. omphalocele, nephrosis, or epidermolysis).

354–356. The answers are: 354-B, 355-A, 356-C. *(Gelehrter, pp 275–283. Thompson, 5/e, pp 411–425.)* The figure that accompanies the question clearly outlines two amniotic cavities indicative of a twin gestation. The single amniotic sample is, thus, representative of only one twin. Because two amnions can occur with either monozygotic or dizygotic twins, zygosity cannot be determined from the ultrasound. Amniotic α-fetoprotein (AFP) fluid values must be correlated with the population mean and gestational age before they are meaningful. Large elevations in AFP fluid values occur with neural tube defects (e.g., anencephaly or spina bifida) and other fetal anomalies that allow leakage of fetal fluids directly into the amniotic fluid. Since spina bifida is a polygenic defect, it is not necessarily concordant (i.e., present in both twins) even if these twins were monozygotic. Sampling of the other amniotic sac would be required before the karyotype and neural tube status of the cotwin could be assessed.

357–361. The answers are: 357-I, 358-G, 359-B, 360-F, 361-E. *(Gelehrter, pp 275–283. Thompson, 5/e, pp 411–425.)* Cerebral palsy has so many causes that prenatal diagnosis is not available. Single birth defects, such as cleft palate, may be detected by ultrasound. People of British or Hispanic ancestry have a high risk for neural tube defects and should be advised of preconceptional folate to lower their risks and of maternal serum α-fetoprotein (MSAFP) as a simple prenatal screen. The early timing of chorionic villus sampling (CVS) provides results before women are visibly pregnant, thus preserving the privacy of their prenatal decisions. A karyotype may be performed on fetuses with anomalies recognized late in pregnancy, using cordocentesis or percutaneous umbilical blood sampling (PUBS). Severe chromosomal diseases, such as trisomy 18, may guide delivery management so as to minimize maternal health risks. Amniocentesis is considered safer than CVS because of more extensive experience with the procedure.

362–364. The answers are: 362-A, 363-C, 364-B. *(Gelehrter, pp 275–283. Thompson, 5/e, pp 411–425.)* Different prenatal diagnostic strategies are available, depending upon the disorder being evaluated. Biochemical disorders, such as Tay-Sachs disease, may be diagnosed by assay of amniocytes or chorionic villi. Recent progress in the molecular characterization of Tay-Sachs mutations makes DNA analysis or hexosaminidase assay feasible. Only DNA analysis is available for cystic fibrosis since the sweat test used for children is not applicable to fetal tissues. Because many different mutations have been described for cystic fibrosis, those present in the parents must be defined for accurate prenatal diagnosis. Although a fetal karyotype is diagnostic for Down syndrome, it only determines sex in fetuses at risk for X-linked disorders when linkage, DNA, or biochemical analyses are not available. The parents are then faced with the difficult decision of terminating a male fetus, knowing that there is a 50 percent chance it is unaffected.

365–367. The answers are: 365-D, 366-B, 367-E. *(Gelehrter, pp 275–283. Thompson, 5/e, pp 411–425.)* All medical procedures must be evaluated in terms of risk-benefit and cost-benefit ratios. Prenatal detection of Down syndrome has been justified based on the savings of dependent care costs, but more optimistic attitudes regarding the potential of Down syndrome children complicate such comparisons. For amniocentesis and chorionic villus sampling (CVS), slightly increased risks for fetal loss above spontaneous abortion rates have been measured in numerous studies. Early CVS may add a slight risk for fetal limb defects. Fetal blood sampling is the most risky prenatal procedure. However, the risks of in vitro fertilization, blastomere sampling for diagnosis by polymerase chain reaction (PCR), and implantation (preimplantation diagnosis) are not known. Pre- and postdiagnostic counseling are essential for good prenatal management, and their absence results in an unknown frequency of inappropriate elective abortions as well as other problems.

Molecular Genetics

DIRECTIONS: Each question below contains four or five suggested responses. Select the **one best** response to each question.

368. The most common type of mutation found in DNA is

(A) insertion
(B) gene deletion
(C) small intragenic deletion
(D) point mutation

369. Single-base substitutions in human DNA have which of the following properties?

(A) They usually result in disease
(B) They are rarely seen in intronic sequences
(C) They usually result in the creation of a new restriction fragment length polymorphism (RFLP)
(D) They may affect transcription
(E) They may result in deletion of a single codon

370. The possible number of sequence combinations for a DNA molecule X bases long is

(A) X
(B) 2X
(C) 4X
(D) 4^x
(E) X^4

371. DNA replication is referred to as being "semiconservative" because

(A) base sequence is conserved
(B) each synthesized DNA molecule has one new strand and one conserved strand
(C) the two DNA strands have complementary sequences
(D) adenine can pair only with thymine
(E) RNA is synthesized from a DNA template

372. In Huntington's disease, patients tend to have an earlier age of onset of symptoms if the gene is inherited from an affected father as opposed to an affected mother. The most likely mechanism for this finding is

(A) mitochondrial inheritance
(B) imprinting
(C) germ-line mosaicism
(D) uniparental disomy
(E) variable expressivity

373. The figure below illustrates a family in which individual I-1 has an autosomal dominant disease. Crossing-over is most likely to have occurred in which of her offspring?

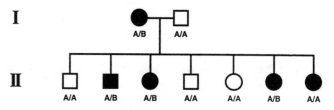

(A) Individual II-1
(B) Individual II-2
(C) Individual II-4
(D) Individual II-6
(E) Individual II-7

374. In the family depicted in the figure below, the genotype of the deceased individual I-1 is most likely to be

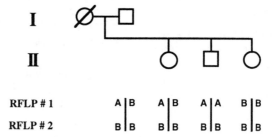

(A) B | B
     B | B
(B) A | B
     B | B
(C) A | A
     B | B
(D) Unable to determine from data

Questions 375–376

Southern blot analysis is performed on DNA from the family depicted below.

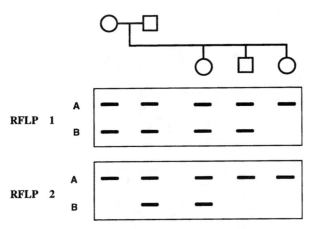

375. The genotype of individual II-2 is

(A) $\begin{array}{c|c} A & B \\ A & B \end{array}$

(B) $\begin{array}{c|c} A & A \\ B & B \end{array}$

(C) $\begin{array}{c|c} B & B \\ A & A \end{array}$

(D) $\begin{array}{c|c} A & B \\ A & A \end{array}$

(E) Unable to determine from the data

376. The genotype of individual I-2 is

A) $\begin{array}{c|c} A & B \\ A & B \end{array}$

B) $\begin{array}{c|c} A & A \\ B & B \end{array}$

C) $\begin{array}{c|c} B & B \\ A & A \end{array}$

D) $\begin{array}{c|c} A & B \\ A & A \end{array}$

E) Unable to determine from the data

Questions 377–379

Prenatal diagnosis is performed for an autosomal dominant condition with onset in adulthood on the family depicted in the figure below. All individuals in generation III are still children. Assume no recombination has occurred.

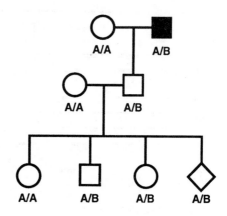

377. What is the status of individual III-4?

(A) Affected
(B) Unaffected
(C) At 50 percent risk
(D) At 25 percent risk
(E) Unable to determine from data

378. What is the status of individual III-1?

(A) Affected
(B) Unaffected
(C) At 50 percent risk
(D) At 25 percent risk
(E) Unable to determine from data

379. Individual II-2 has begun to show signs and symptoms of the disorder. With this information in mind, what is the status of the fetus?

(A) Affected
(B) Unaffected
(C) At 50 percent risk
(D) At 25 percent risk
(E) Unable to determine from data

Questions 380–381

A couple comes to the physician's office after having had a child with cystic fibrosis. The wife is now pregnant, and the couple desires a prenatal diagnosis. Amniocentesis is performed at 17 weeks of pregnancy, and the results are shown in the figure below. Assume that no recombination has occurred.

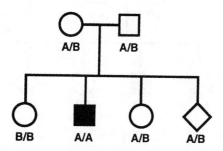

380. What is the status of the fetus (II-4)?

(A) Affected
(B) Unaffected, carrier
(C) Unaffected, noncarrier
(D) Unable to determine from the data

381. What is the status of individual II-1?

(A) Affected
(B) Unaffected, carrier
(C) Unaffected, noncarrier
(D) Unable to determine from the data

Questions 382–383

Prenatal diagnosis is performed for an autosomal recessive condition. Results are shown in the figure below. Assume that no recombination has oc-curred.

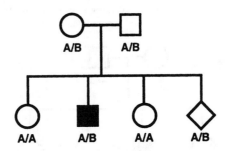

382. What is the status of the fetus (II-4)?

(A) Affected
(B) Unaffected, carrier
(C) Unaffected, noncarrier
(D) Unable to determine from the data

383. What is the status of individual II-1?

(A) Affected
(B) Unaffected, carrier
(C) Unaffected, noncarrier
(D) Unable to determine from the data

---

384. What is the complementary strand to the normal DNA sequence 5′ CAC TGG 3′?

(A) 3′ CAC TGG 5′
(B) 3′ ACA GTT 5′
(C) 3′ GTG ACC 5′
(D) 5′ GGT CAC 3′
(E) 5′ GTG ACC 3′

385. What is the corresponding messenger RNA for the normal DNA sequence 5′ CAC TGG 3′?

(A) 5′ CAC TGG 3′
(B) 3′ CAC UGG 5′
(C) 5′ GUG ACC 3′
(D) 3′ GUG ACC 5′
(E) 5′ GGU CAC 3′

Questions 386–387

A candidate gene is being evaluated for linkage with the disorder pseudoachondroplasia, a relatively common skeletal dysplasia. DNA is obtained from members of a 3-generation family, and Southern blot analysis is performed. The results are shown below.

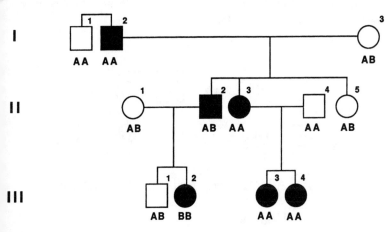

386. Which of the following individuals are affected with pseudo-achondroplasia?

A) I-2, II-2, III-2
B) I-1, II-2, III-2
C) I-1, II-1, III-1
D) I-2, II-3, II-4
E) II-2, II-3, II-4

387. Linkage of the pseudoachondroplasia gene to this candidate gene is ex-cluded because

A) individual II-2 and II-3 are both affected and have different genotypes
B) individual II-2 transmitted the B allele from his unaffected mother (I-3) to his affected daughter (III-2)
C) individual II-2, who is affected, and his sister (II-5), who is unaffected, have the same genotype
D) individual II-2 transmitted the A allele from his affected father to his un-affected son (III-1)
E) no conclusions about linkage can be drawn from this Southern blot

Questions 388–389

A family with the autosomal dominant nail-patella syndrome (abnormal nails, patella, and other bones) requests evaluation. Individual II-3 in the figure below, who is affected with nail-patella syndrome, wants to know if prenatal diagnosis is possible for future pregnancies. Because the ABO blood group locus is known to be linked to the nail-patella locus on chromosome 9, blood typing was performed on the family.

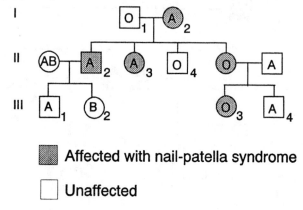

▨ Affected with nail-patella syndrome

☐ Unaffected

388. Which of the following individuals gives evidence of a crossover between the ABO and nail-patella loci?
(A) Individual II-2
(B) Individual II-4
(C) Individual II-5
(D) Individual III-1
(E) Individual III-4

389. Because of the 10 percent recombination frequency between ABO and nail-patella loci, individual II-2 in the figure requested more definitive testing to allow a prenatal diagnosis. Among the testing possibilities listed below, which would be most likely to provide a definitive prenatal diagnosis?
(A) Use of a variable number of tandem repeats (VNTR) near the ABO locus for linkage analysis of the family
(B) Cloning of the nail-patella gene and screening of skin fibroblasts from individual II-3 by Northern analysis
(C) Use of new restriction fragment length polymorphism (RFLP) less than 1 centimorgan (cM) from the nail-patella locus for linkage analysis of the family
(D) Cloning of the nail-patella gene and screening for altered gene restriction fragments by Southern analysis
(E) Cloning of the nail-patella gene and screening for altered gene fragment mobility by single-strand conformational polymorphism (SSCP) analysis

390. The family with autosomal dominant nail-patella syndrome is investigated using a new restriction fragment length polymorphism (RFLP) on chromosome 9 that is less than 1 centimorgan (cM) from the nail-patella locus. The figure below shows a diagrammatic Southern blot beneath the family pedigree with larger (1) and smaller (2) polymorphic fragments. These fragments derive from the polymorphism of the restriction enzyme site, E_2 (*bottom*). When the E_2 site is absent, the DNA probe used for Southern analysis (*thick bar*) detects the larger fragment 1 as diagrammed. For individual II-2 (genotype 1,2) to have a prenatal diagnosis of a fetus with nail-patella syndrome, her husband must have which of the following RFLP genotypes?

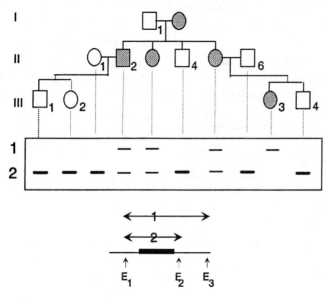

(A) 1,1 or 2,2
(B) 1,2
(C) 2,2
(D) 1,1
(E) 1,1 or 2,2 or 1,2

391. Deletions of 11p13 may result in Wilms tumor, aniridia, genitourinary malformations, and mental retardation—that is, the WAGR syndrome. In some patients, however, not all features are seen. Additionally, individual features of this syndrome may be inherited separately in a Mendelian fashion. Limited features may be seen in patients without visible chromosomal deletions. The most likely mechanism for this finding is

(A) mitochondrial inheritance
(B) imprinting
(C) germ-line mosaicism
(D) uniparental disomy
(E) contiguous gene syndrome

392. The average number of recombination events per chromosome per meiosis is

(A) < 1
(B) 1 to 3
(C) 5 to 10
(D) 50
(E) 100

393. In Leber's hereditary optic neuropathy, all individuals are related through the maternal line. Affected males cannot pass on the disease. The most likely mechanism for this finding is

(A) mitochondrial inheritance
(B) imprinting
(C) germ-line mosaicism
(D) uniparental disomy
(E) variable expressivity

394. If θ (theta) is the recombination fraction for two different DNA fragments, then random assortment is represented by

(A) $\theta = 0.0$
(B) $\theta = 0.01$
(C) $\theta = 0.1$
(D) $\theta = 0.5$
(E) $\theta = 1.0$

DIRECTIONS: Each numbered question or incomplete statement below is NEGATIVELY phrased. Select the **one best** lettered response.

395. All the following statements regarding in situ hybridization are true EXCEPT

(A) DNA probes are annealed to metaphase chromosomes
(B) the method is useful for both single-copy and repetitive DNA sequences
(C) chromosomes are spread on a slide and denatured in place
(D) probes may be labeled with fluorescent material
(E) exact localization of genes is possible

396. All the following statements regarding the Human Genome Project are true EXCEPT

(A) it represents a national effort
(B) it involves constructing physical and genetic linkage maps
(C) it includes plans to sequence all genes
(D) maps are maintained in a computer data base, which is available to all interested parties

397. Repetitive sequences in DNA include all the following EXCEPT

(A) L1 family (LINES)
(B) Alu sequences
(C) alphoid sequences
(D) fragile sites
(E) satellite DNA

398. All the following statements regarding somatic cell hybrids are true EXCEPT

(A) individual hybrid cells are useful to map genes
(B) human cells are fused to mouse or hamster cells
(C) many human chromosomes are lost
(D) regional mapping is possible when only fragments of chromosomes are present
(E) human chromosomes and rodent chromosomes may be distinguished cytogenetically

399. All the following statements regarding immunoglobulins are true EXCEPT

(A) a large number of antibodies are encoded by a relatively small number of genes
(B) each immunoglobulin molecule contains two identical heavy chains and two identical light chains
(C) genes encoding heavy and light chains are linked
(D) the five different classes of immunoglobulins differ in their heavy chains
(E) variable regions determine antibody specificity

400. DNA from normal individuals was digested with a restriction endonuclease and hybridized with probe A. The Southern blot obtained is seen below. All the following statements regarding this Southern blot are true EXCEPT

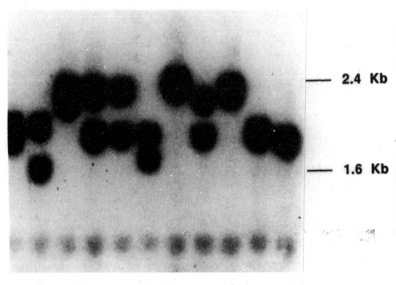

(A) multiple alleles are present within this segment of DNA
(B) blots such as these are used to determine allele frequencies
(C) alleles range in size from 1.6 to 2.4 kb
(D) more than one gene is present within this segment of DNA
(E) patients who are both homozygous and heterozygous are seen

---

401. All the following statements regarding logarithm of the odds (lod) scores are true EXCEPT

(A) a lod score is the log (to base 10) of the odds in favor of linkage
(B) the higher the lod score, the more likely that there is linkage
(C) lod scores determine the relative positions of multiple DNA fragments
(D) lod scores may be determined for different recombination fractions

402. All the following statements concerning mitochondrial DNA are correct EXCEPT

(A) it is double-stranded
(B) it encodes its own set of transfer RNAs (tRNAs)
(C) it encodes 13 proteins translated within the nucleus
(D) it is inherited from the mother
(E) most encoded proteins function in oxidative phosphorylation

403. The "genetic code" stores information that determines the amino acid sequence of proteins. All the following statements regarding the genetic code are true EXCEPT

(A) information is stored as sets of three adjacent bases
(B) the code is degenerate (i.e., more than one codon may exist for a single amino acid)
(C) in most cases, the code is universal (i.e., codons are the same in all organisms)
(D) there are 64 codons, all of which code for amino acids
(E) the sequence of codons on a DNA molecule corresponds to the sequence of amino acids in the complimentary polypeptide chain

404. Sickle cell anemia is caused by a point mutation in the hemoglobin gene, resulting in the substitution of a single amino acid in the mature protein. This mutation could be detected by all the following methods EXCEPT

(A) allele-specific oligonucleotide (ASO) hybridization
(B) Southern blot analysis
(C) DNA sequencing
(D) polymerase chain reaction (PCR) with restriction enzyme digestion
(E) Western blot analysis

DIRECTIONS: Each group of questions below consists of lettered headings followed by a set of numbered items. For each numbered item select the **one** lettered heading with which it is **most** closely associated. Each lettered heading may be used **once, more than once or not at all.**

Questions 405–407

Match each of the following techniques with the specific use for which it is known.

(A) Detects specific base pairs
(B) Detects DNA molecules
(C) Detects RNA molecules
(D) Detects proteins
(E) Determines chromosome structure

405. Southern blot analysis

406. Northern blot analysis

407. Western blot analysis

Questions 408–410

Match the terms below with their approximate DNA contents.

(A) 1000 bp
(B) 40,000 bp
(C) 2×10^6 bp
(D) 1.5×10^8 bp
(E) 3×10^9 bp

408. Average chromosome

409. Average chromosome band from high-resolution karyotype

410. Average-sized gene

Questions 411–412

Match the descriptions below with the appropriate method of DNA analysis.

(A) Polymerase chain reaction (PCR)
(B) Allele-specific oligonucleotide (ASO) hybridization
(C) Pulsed-field gel electrophoresis
(D) Agarose gel electrophoresis
(E) Chromosome walking

411. Rapidly amplifies fragments of DNA

412. Allows separation of relatively long sequences of DNA (up to > 5000 kb)

Questions 413–414

Match each of the following terms with its partial definition.

(A) Determines site of initiation of transcription
(B) A cryptic splice site
(C) At the 3′ end of mRNA
(D) Located in an intron

413. Promoter region

414. Polyadenylation site

Questions 415–417

Match each of the following terms with its partial definition.

(A) Structure to which spindle fibers attach
(B) Proteins, rich in basic amino acids, that are packaged with DNA in chromosomes
(C) Condensed packages of proteins and DNA
(D) Primary constriction
(E) Point of attachment for sister chromatids

415. Histones

416. Chromatin

417. Heterochromatin

Questions 418–420

Match each of the following terms with its partial definition.

(A) Pyrimidine
(B) Purine
(C) Pairs with guanine
(D) Sugar
(E) Nucleotide

418. Deoxyribose

419. Adenine

420. Thymine

Questions 421–423

The hypothetical "stimulin" gene contains two exons that encode a protein of 100 amino acids. They are separated by an intron of 100 bp beginning after the codon for amino acid 10. Stimulin messenger RNA (mRNA) has 5' and 3' untranslated regions of 70 and 30 nucleotides, respectively. Match the characteristics of the stimulin gene with the appropriate measures.

(A) 500 bp
(B) 400 bp
(C) 300 bp
(D) 100 bp
(E) 70 bp

421. Size of mature stimulin RNA minus residual poly(A)

422. Smallest stimulin gene

423. Distance of first splice site from transcription start site

Questions 424–426

Match each of the following terms with its partial definition.

(A) Conversion of triplet codons into amino acids
(B) Duplication of DNA
(C) Pairing of complimentary strands of nucleic acids
(D) Conversion of DNA to RNA
(E) Conversion of RNA to DNA

424. Replication

425. Translation

426. Transcription

Questions 427–429

The family with the autosomal dominant nail-patella syndrome (questions 388–389 and 390) required a second evaluation because individual II-3 could not have a prenatal diagnosis using new restriction fragment length polymorphisms (RFLPs) based on her husband's genotype. The figure below illustrates a polymerase chain reaction (PCR) analysis that examines a variable number of tandem repeats (VNTRs) in a DNA region very near the nail-patella locus. Each repeat contains two nucleotides, and the number of repeats varies to produce at least six differently sized alleles when the region is amplified by PCR, using primers P_1 and P_2. Based on the family analysis shown in the figure, match the individuals below with the correct genotype.

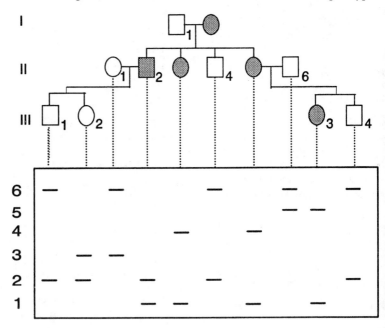

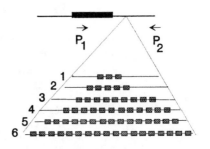

(A) DNA analysis not shown
(B) 2,6
(C) 3,6
(D) 1,4
(E) 1,5

427. Individual III-1

428. Individual II-3

429. Individual I-1

Questions 430–432

Analysis of the family with nail-patella syndrome by variable number of tandem repeats (VNTRs) shown in the figure that accompanies the previous question allows several of the females to select the option of prenatal diagnosis. Ignoring the possibility of crossovers, match the matings listed below with the fetal results.

(A) Fetal genotype 1,4—50 percent chance of being affected
(B) Fetal genotype 1,2—non-paternity
(C) Fetal genotype 4,4—50 percent chance of being affected
(D) Fetal genotype 2,5—unaffected fetus
(E) Fetal genotype 1,4—100 percent chance of being affected

430. Individual II-3 with a man of genotype 2,4

431. Individual II-5 with a man of genotype 1,5

432. Individual III-3 with a man of genotype 2,3

Questions 433–435

Match each of the following altered amino acid sequences with the type of DNA mutation most likely to be responsible for it, given the following normal amino acid chain:
Cys→Gly→Gly→Ser→Met→Val

(A) Missense mutations
(B) Nonsense mutations
(C) Frameshift mutations
(D) Deletions
(E) Insertions

433. Cys→Gly→Ser→Met→Val

434. Cys→Gly→Gly

435. Cys→Gly→Glu→Ser→Met→Val

Questions 436–437

Match each of the terms below with its partial definition.

(A) A recombinant DNA molecule that contains a DNA sequence of interest
(B) The DNA molecule into which the DNA sequence of interest is cloned
(C) Labeled DNA or RNA fragment used for hybridization
(D) Oligonucleotide designed to detect a particular allele
(E) Oligonucleotide designed for DNA sequencing or polymerase chain reactions (PCRs)

436. Probe

437. Primer

Questions 438–439

Match each of the following terms with its partial definition.

(A) Tumor suppressor gene
(B) Responsible for unregulated cell growth and proliferation (i.e., tumor development)
(C) Codes for any RNA or protein product
(D) Regulates gene expression, especially in development
(E) Products provide basic functions

438. Homeobox gene

439. Housekeeping gene

Questions 440–441

Match each of the following terms with its partial definition.

(A) Intergenic DNA
(B) Removed in processing of RNA
(C) Coding region of DNA
(D) Located in the upstream flanking region of DNA
(E) Closely resemble genes but are nonfunctional

440. Intron

441. Exon

Questions 442–444

A sister and brother present with mental retardation and connective tissue laxity. A karyotype on the brother is positive for the fragile X marker, and DNA analysis is performed on the family as shown in the figure below. The analysis demonstrates amplified DNA fragments obtained by the polymerase chain reaction (PCR) and separated by size on a polyacrylamide gel. Primers for the PCR reaction span the fragile X region that contains variable numbers of trinucleotide repeats. These repeats vary between 6 to 52 copies for normal people, 52 to 230 for asymptomatic female carriers, and up to 1000 for affected males or symptomatic female carriers. The *dark bands* represent discretely sized fragments, while the *grey bands* represent smears of multiply sized fragments. With reference to the diagram, match each of the individuals below with the descriptions that are most appropriate.

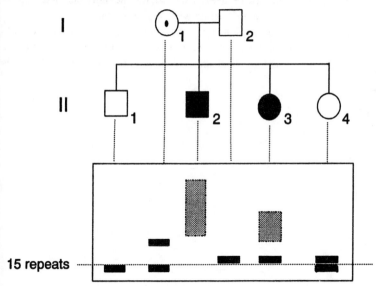

(A) One DNA fragment with repeat number in normal range
(B) Two DNA fragments with repeat numbers in normal range
(C) Two DNA fragments—one with repeat numbers typical of asymptomatic female carriers, another in normal range
(D) Smear of multiply sized DNA fragments only
(E) Smear of multiply sized DNA fragments, plus one DNA fragment with repeat numbers in normal range

442. Individual I-1

443. Individual II-3

444. Individual II-2

Questions 445–447

Referring again to the polymerase chain reaction (PCR) analysis shown in the previous question, match each of the individual DNA analyses below with the explanation that best describes it.

    (A) A "premutation," representing moderate amplification of triplet repeats, is present in an asymptomatic individual who has a 25 percent risk of having a child with fragile X syndrome

    (B) A "premutation," representing moderate amplification of triplet repeats, is present in an asymptomatic individual who has virtually no risk of having a child with fragile X syndrome

    (C) No repeat amplification has occurred, and the individual has virtually no risk of having a child with fragile X syndrome

    (D) No repeat amplification has occurred, but the individual has a 25 percent risk of having a child with fragile X syndrome

    (E) Dramatic amplification and instability of triplet repeats has occurred with mosaicism for different repeat lengths in different tissue types, leading to a broad smear of fragment sizes after PCR analysis

445. Individual II-3

446. Individual I-1

447. Individual II-4

Questions 448–451

Gyrate atrophy is a relatively rare recessive genetic disorder caused by a deficiency of ornithine aminotransferase. Affected individuals have progressive chorioretinal degeneration. The gene for ornithine aminotransferase has been cloned, its structure determined, and mutations in affected individuals have been extensively studied. Match the following possible results of molecular and enzymatic testing with the explanations listed below.

(A) Point mutation in noncoding region
(B) 2 kb deletion
(C) 2 kb insertion
(D) Deletion of entire gene
(E) Nonsense mutation
(F) Missense mutation
(G) Small in-frame deletion

448. Normal Southern blot; absent enzymatic activity

449. Abnormal Southern blot (altered restriction pattern); normal enzymatic activity

450. Northern blotting shows messenger RNA (mRNA) normal size; no enzymatic activity

451. Normal Southern blot; Northern blotting shows absent mRNA

Questions 452–454

The DNA sequence below is a portion of exon 8 of the ornithine trans-carbamylase gene beginning with amino acid residue 208.

Normal: 5' AAT GGT ACC AAG CTG TTG CTG ACA 3'

Match the statements below with the mutant sequences, using the following genetic and amino acid codes:

Asparagine (Asn): AAT   Leucine (Leu): CTG, TTG
Glycine (Gly): GGT   Phenylalanine (Phe): TTC
Threonine (Thr): ACC, ACA   Stop codon: TCA, TTA, CTA
Lysine (Lys): AAG

  (A) 5'AAT GGT ACC AAG TTG CTG ACA 3'
  (B) 5'AAT GGT ACC AAG CTA TTG CTG ACA 3'
  (C) 5'AAT GGT ACC AAG TTG TTG CTG ACA 3'
  (D) 5'AAT GGT ACC AAG CTG TTC CTG ACA 3'
  (E) 5'AAT GGT ACC AAG CTG TTG CTA CA 3'

452. Leucine → phenylalanine at position 213

453. Chain termination following amino acid residue 211

454. Chain termination following amino acid residue 213

Molecular Genetics
Answers

368. The answer is D. *(Gelehrter, pp 21–23. Thompson, 5/e, pp 115–140.)* A mutation is a permanent change in DNA. Multiple types of mutations can occur. The most common type of mutation is a *point mutation* in which a single nucleotide is replaced. Point mutations may be silent and, therefore, not affect the final polypeptide product. They may also be *missense mutations,* which cause a single amino acid change; *nonsense mutations,* which cause a premature "stop" in DNA transcription; mutations that alter RNA splicing; or mutations that alter the regulation of transcription.

369. The answer is D. *(Gelehrter, pp 21–23. Thompson, 5/e, pp 115–141.)* Most DNA variation is normal (DNA polymorphisms). A very small percentage of changes cause disease. Variations in DNA occur approximately every 100 to 200 nucleotides in introns and flanking DNA. Frequently these changes cannot be detected by restriction enzymes and, therefore, do not result in the formation of a new restriction fragment length polymorphism (RFLP). Point mutations do not delete entire codons but may affect their transcription by altering promoter or enhancer sites.

370. The answer is D. *(Gelehrter, p 11. Thompson, 5/e, p 46.)* At any one position along a DNA molecule, four possibilities exist (A, T, C, and G); therefore, for a sequence X bases long, there are 4^x combinations. This allows for a nearly infinite number of combinations of codons and amino acid sequences to be stored in our genetic material.

371. The answer is B. *(Thompson, 5/e, p 11.)* DNA is a double-stranded molecule. As the DNA double helix unwinds, each individual strand serves as a template for replication. This allows for the formation of two new double-stranded molecules, each of which contains a conserved strand of DNA along with a newly formed complementary strand. Because only one strand of the new DNA molecule is a conserved strand, the process is referred to as "semi-conservative."

372. The answer is B. *(Thompson, 5/e, p 92.)* Imprinting is a phenomenon in which the sex of the transmitting parent may affect the expression of the gene (the phenotype). These differences appear to be associated with differences in methylation patterns of DNA.

373. The answer is E. *(Gelehrter, pp 202–207. Thompson, 5/e, pp 178–190.)* In the pedigree that accompanies the question, all affected individuals appear to have inherited the paternal B allele, whereas unaffected individuals have inherited the paternal A allele. The sole exception to this is individual II-7 who inherited both the disease gene and the paternal A allele. If the polymorphism studied is linked to the disease gene, individual II-7 must be a recombinant in whom crossing-over has occurred between the polymorphism and the disease gene. To definitively prove linkage, more families need to be studied.

374. The answer is B. *(Gelehrter, pp 202–207. Thompson, 5/e, pp 178–190.)* In the example in the question, phase (i.e., those alleles that travel together) has already been determined. Individual II-2 has inherited two chromosomes, each of which contain the AB haplotype. Therefore, each parent must have one chromosome that contains the AB haplotype. Similarly, individual II-3 has the BB haplotype on both chromosomes, which implies that each parent must have one chromosome that carries the BB haplotype. The genotype of the deceased individual I-1 can now be deduced as AB/BB.

375–376. The answers are: 375-D, 376-A. *(Gelehrter, pp 202–207. Thompson, 5/e, pp 178–190.)* In the example in the questions, phase (i.e., those alleles that travel together) must be determined. Individual II-2 is homozygous for allele A at restriction fragment length polymorphism (RFLP) number 2. Therefore, his genotype must be AA/BA. The mother in the family, individual I-1, is homozygous for the A allele at RFLP 2. Therefore, her genotype is AA/AB. Using the same logic, genotypes for individual II-2 (AA/BA) and individual II-3 (AA/AA) may be determined. Since individual II-3 must have inherited one chromosome from each parent, the father must have one chromosome containing the haplotype AA. His other chromosome must, therefore, contain the haplotype BB.

377–379. The answers are: 377-C, 378-B, 379-A. *(Gelehrter, pp 202–207. Thompson, 5/e, pp 178–190.)* Individual II-2 has inherited the A allele from his mother (since she is homozygous for this allele) and the B allele from his father, the affected individual. In turn, he has passed on this B allele to the fetus, individual III-4. Since it is not known which grandpaternal allele is linked to the disease, and individual II-2 may be too young to be showing any signs or symptoms of the disease, we can only say that the fetus is at the same risk as his father—that is, 50 percent.

Individual III-1 has inherited the A allele from her father. Assuming that no recombination has occurred, individual III-1 is unaffected.

Individual II-2 has inherited the B allele from his father. Since he is now showing evidence of the disorder, it can be determined that this B allele is linked to the disease gene. The fetus, individual III-4, has inherited this B allele from his father. Therefore, assuming no recombination, the fetus must be affected.

380–381. The answers are: 380-B, 381-C. *(Gelehrter, pp 202–207. Thompson, 5/e, pp 178–190.)* Cystic fibrosis, the commonest autosomal recessive disorder among Caucasians, affects the lungs and the exocrine pancreas. The proband in the pedigree that accompanies the question (individual II-2) has inherited the A allele from each parent. The fetus has inherited one A allele, which is linked to the disease, and one B allele, which is not linked to the disease. Therefore, the fetus is a carrier of cystic fibrosis but is not affected with the disease.

Because the proband in the pedigree (individual II-2) inherited the A allele from each parent, the A allele must be linked to the disease gene in both parents. Individual II-1 has inherited the B allele from each parent and is, therefore, unaffected and a noncarrier of the disease gene.

382–383. The answers are: 382-D, 383-B. *(Gelehrter, pp 202–207. Thompson, 5/e, pp 178–190.)* In the case presented in the question, the affected individual (II-2) inherited the A allele from one parent and the B allele from the other. However, it cannot be determined which allele came from which parent. The fetus has also inherited the AB genotype; however, it cannot be determined which allele came from which parent. Therefore, the disease status of the fetus cannot be determined.

Individual II-1 has inherited the AA genotype. Since she has inherited an A allele from both parents, it can be determined that one of those two alleles must be linked to the disease gene, although it cannot be determined from which parent it was inherited. The other A allele is not linked to the disease gene. The individual is, therefore, an unaffected carrier of this autosomal recessive condition.

384. The answer is C. *(Gelehrter, pp 11–12. Thompson, 5/e, pp 32–33.)* The DNA molecule is a double helix composed of two complementary strands, often called the "sense" and the "antisense" strand. Hydrogen bonds between the two strands can form between the A and the T or the C and the G. One strand runs 5′ to 3′, while the complementary strand runs 3′ to 5′. Therefore, in this case, the complementary strands must be:

5′ CAC TGG 3′
3′ GTG ACC 5′

385. The answer is D. *(Gelehrter, pp 13–15. Thompson, 5/e, pp 44–47.)* Transcription begins at the 3′ end of the DNA template. Corresponding bases are added to the RNA molecule in the 5′ to 3′ direction. Additionally, the base thymine is replaced in RNA by uracil. Following these rules, the messenger RNA (mRNA) formed in this case would be:

DNA: 5′ CAC TGG 3′
mRNA: 3′ GUG ACC 5′

386–387. The answers are: 386-A, 387-B. *(Gelehrter, pp 202–207. Thompson, 5/e, pp 195–196.)* Affected individuals are denoted by solid symbols. In this pedigree, there are many affected individuals including I-2, II-2, II-3, III-2, III-3, and III-4.

The candidate gene approach has been used in the mapping of many different disorders. Cloned genes are selected that are believed to have a role in the pathophysiology of that disorder. In this case, the gene being evaluated cannot be responsible for the disorder because individual II-2 has passed the B allele from his unaffected mother to his affected daughter. The disorder and the candidate gene do not cosegregate. In the case of individual III-1, it is impossible to determine which parent has transmitted which allele since both parents are heterozygous. In evaluating linkage, one cannot look at the genotype in isolation. Two individuals may have the same genotype but may have inherited the alleles from different parents. It is important to remember that the polymorphism being evaluated is a marker for the disease and not the disease itself.

388–389. The answers are: 388-C, 389-E. *(Gelehrter, pp 193–228. Thompson, 5/e, pp 115–142.)* The affected individual I-2 in the figure that accompanies the question establishes phase for the two loci in that the A blood group allele is present on the same number 9 chromosome as is the abnormal nail-patella allele. Affected individuals II-2 and II-3 have inherited this A allele and, as expected, the abnormal nail-patella allele. Individual II-5 has inherited the O blood group allele from her mother, yet she is affected with nail-patella syndrome. Transmission of the abnormal nail-patella allele and the O blood group allele to her daughter (III-3) establishes that a crossover occurred in individual II-5.

Linkage analysis requires several affected and unaffected family members to establish phase of marker and disease loci, sufficient polymorphism of the marker to be informative, and the ability to detect the marker in fetal cells.

Variable number of tandem repeat (VNTR) markers usually have more alleles and, thus, are preferred for linkage studies over restriction fragment length polymorphisms (RFLPs). However, the proximity of the marker to the disease locus is most important, as crossovers occur at a frequency of about 1 percent for each centimorgan (cM) of genetic distance. More accurate than indirect genetic linkage methods are physical methods that directly examine gene structure. Northern analysis to show decreased mRNA expression, Southern analysis to demonstrate gene deletions via altered restriction fragments, and single-strand conformational polymorphism (SSCP) analysis to demonstrate deletions or point mutations in the gene provide increasing sensitivity for the range of possible gene mutations. Because point mutations are more frequent than mutations ablating expression or gene deletions, SSCP would be the most sensitive.

390. The answer is C. *(Gelehrter, pp 193–228. Thompson, 5/e, pp 115–142.)* Restriction fragment length polymorphisms (RFLPs) provide a limited number of variant alleles for linkage studies. In the figure that accompanies the question, two differently sized DNA fragments result from digestion of patient DNA with restriction enzyme E based on the variable presence of restriction site E_2. It can be seen from the pedigree that the larger DNA fragment allele (1) segregates with the nail-patella allele. Note the absence of crossovers since this RFLP locus is less than 1 centimorgan (cM) away from the nail-patella locus (less than 1 percent crossover frequency). For individual II-3 to have a prenatal diagnosis, it must be possible to examine fetal DNA for the presence of allele 1 and know that, if present, it is derived from the mother. Thus, the paternal genotype must be 2,2. Note, the thicker bands in the Southern blot represent homozygous 2,2 genotypes that yield signals of double density.

391. The answer is E. *(Thompson, 5/e, pp 87–88.)* Contiguous gene syndromes, also known as microdeletion syndromes, occur when deletions result in the loss of several different closely linked loci. Depending on the size of the deletion, different phenotypes may result. Mutations in the individual genes may result in isolated features that may be inherited in a Mendelian fashion.

392. The answer is B. *(Gelehrter, pp 19–20. Thompson, 5/e, pp 178–180.)* Crossing-over is the breaking and rejoining of two homologous chromosomes, which occurs in meiotic prophase I. This results in the recombination of genetic material creating a new chromosome that contains portions from both of the parental chromosomes. The average number of crossovers per chromosome per meiosis is one to three.

393.   The answer is A. *(Gelehrter, pp 44. Thompson, 5/e, pp 89–90.)* Mitochondrial inheritance is the transmission of genes encoded on the mitochondrial genome; Mendelian inheritance is the transmission of genes encoded on the nuclear genome. Mitochondria, located in the cytoplasm of cells, are maternally transmitted; therefore, any disorder coded for on the mitochondrial genome is transmitted through the maternal line only. Affected males cannot pass on the disorder. Unlike X-linked recessive disorders, equal numbers of males and females are affected.

394.   The answer is D. *(Gelehrter, pp 205–207. Thompson, 5/e, pp 183–185.)* The recombination fraction denoted by θ (theta) is the fraction of meioses during which recombination takes place. When the recombination fraction is 0, no recombination has taken place. However, when the recombination fraction is 0.5, recombination has taken place 50 percent of the time. This implies that recombination is a completely random event (random assortment) and that the two loci are not linked.

395.   The answer is E. *(Gelehrter, pp 195–196. Thompson, 5/e, p 175.)* In situ hybridization is a technique that is used for gene mapping. Metaphase chromosomes are denatured in place (in situ) on a slide. DNA probes, which may be labeled with radioactive or fluorescent material, are then annealed to the DNA. This method can be used to map genes with a resolution of 1 to 2 million base pairs. However, since this is still substantially larger than most genes, exact localization is not possible.

396.   The answer is A. *(Gelehrter, pp 289–292. Thompson, 5/e, p 186.)* The Human Genome Project is an international effort to map and sequence all of the genes in the human genome. Physical and genetic linkage maps are being constructed of all 23 pairs of human chromosomes. In the United States, the project was initially headed by James Watson who, along with Francis Crick, originally described the structure of the DNA double helix. All current mapping data are maintained on-line on a continually edited computer data base.

397.   The answer is D. *(Gelehrter, p 71. Thompson, 5/e, pp 38–39.)* Approximately 10 percent of the genome consists of highly repetitive, clustered sequences of DNA organized in tandem arrays. These regions of DNA, collectively called *satellite DNAs,* include alphoid sequences and tend to be located in specific regions, such as centromeres and telomeres. Approximately 15 percent of the genome consists of other repetitive sequences of DNA, which are scattered throughout the regions of single-copy DNA. These repetitive DNA families include the Alu family and the L1 family (or LINES).

398. The answer is A. *(Gelehrter, p 197–198. Thompson, 5/e, pp 169–173.)* Somatic cell hybridization is a method of gene mapping that involves the process of fusing human cells to mouse or hamster cells. During this process, each cell may lose many of its human chromosomes yet retain its rodent cells. Clonal hybrid lines are prepared, and panels of these lines are used to map specific genes. Since rodent and human chromosomes can be differentiated cytogentically, it is possible to determine which human chromosomes are present in each cell line. Southern blots are prepared, using the DNA fragment to be mapped. Each lane of the blot represents a different hybrid line. It can then be deduced which specific human chromosome is present in all the lines in which the DNA fragment is present. Regional mapping can be done similarly, using hybrid lines that contain only fragments of human chromosomes.

399. The answer is C. *(Gelehrter, pp 93–94. Thompson, 5/e, pp 342–344.)* Immunoglobulins are formed by a unique process in which a small number of genes code for a nearly infinite number of antibodies. Immunoglobulin molecules contain two identical heavy (H) and two identical light (L) chains. The genes for these chains are located in regions on three separate chromosomes and, therefore, are not linked. H and L chains contain constant and variable regions. The five classes of immunoglobulins (i.e., IgA, IgE, IgG, IgM, and IgD) differ in their H-chain constant regions. It is the variable regions that determine antibody specificity.

400. The answer is D. *(Gelehrter, pp 78–82. Thompson, 5/e, pp 106–108.)* Although many DNA probes detect only two different alleles, some regions of DNA are more highly polymorphic. The results of Southern blot analysis may be a multiple allele system as is seen in the figure that accompanies the question. According to the labeling on this blot, these alleles range in size from 1.6 to 2.4 kb. By analyzing DNA from large groups of ethnically diverse individuals, the frequency of various alleles within the normal population can be determined. These statistics are useful in evaluating linkage disequilibrium in which certain alleles are disproportionately linked with other alleles. Because each lane contains DNA from both chromosomes of each individual, those with a single band are noted to be homozygous at this site and those with two bands are heterozygous. Although multiple alleles are noted on this blot, no conclusions can be drawn with regard to the specific content of the genetic material evaluated (i.e., the number of genes).

401. The answer is C. *(Gelehrter, pp 205–206. Thompson, 5/e, pp 183–185.)* A *lo*garithm of the *od*ds (lod) score is a statistical method used to evaluate the likelihood that two loci are linked. It is the $\log_{10}$ of the odds of linkage. Positive values imply linkage, while negative values imply that the loci are not linked. By convention, linkage is said to be proven when the lod score is ≥ 3 and disproven when it is ≤ -2. Lod scores can be determined for different recombination fractions with the maximum lod score indicating the likely frequency of recombination. Lod scores by themselves do not allow the ordering of different loci along the chromosome.

402. The answer is C. *(Gelehrter, p 44. Thompson, 5/e, pp 89–90.)* Mitochondrial DNA is a double-stranded, closed, circular molecule of 16,569 base pairs. It encodes its own transfer RNAs (tRNAs) and encodes 13 proteins involved with oxidative phosphorylation, which are translated within the mitochondrion. The mitochondrion are inherited from the mother.

403. The answer is D. *(Gelehrter, p 15. Thompson, 5/e, pp 46–47.)* The "genetic code" uses three base "words," or codons, to specify the 20 different amino acids. Since there are four nucleotides that can be arrayed in 2^4 or 64 different combinations, the code must be degenerate with more than one codon for a single amino acid. Sixty-one codons code for amino acids; three codons are "stop" codons and result in chain termination. The genetic code is universal with codons coding for the same amino acids in all organisms.

404. The answer is E. *(Gelehrter, pp 76–88, 102–106. Thompson, 5/e, pp 106–113.)* Sickle cell anemia is an autosomal recessive hemoglobinopathy that occurs in approximately 1 in 500 births in the African-American population. It is caused by a single nucleotide substitution in codon 6 of the hemoglobin gene. This mutation abolishes a restriction site for the enzyme MstII and, thus, can be detected by Southern blot analysis after digestion with this enzyme. It can similarly be detected when a polymerase chain reaction (PCR) product is digested with this enzyme. Allele-specific oligonucleotide (ASO) hybridization also detects single, base-pair substitutions. DNA sequencing detects any change in the order of bases in a DNA fragment. Western blotting is a technique that examines the size and amount of mutant protein in cell extracts and, therefore, would not identify the sickle cell mutation in DNA.

405–407. The answers are: 405-B, 406-C, 407-D. *(Gelehrter, pp 76–88. Thompson, 5/e, pp 105–112.)* Southern blotting is a technique that was first described by Edward Southern. DNA fragments are separated on agarose gels by electrophoresis and then transferred to nitrocellulose filters. The filters are then exposed to labeled probes, which hybridize to the DNA fragments. Northern blotting is an analogous procedure, which allows for the detection of RNA fragments. Western blotting is a technique used for detecting proteins, usually using immunologic methods.

408–410. The answers are: 408-D, 409-C, 410-B. *(Gelehrter, pp 69–129. Thompson, 5/e, pp 97–114.)* The 6×10^9 bp of DNA in each human diploid cell is apportioned among 46 chromosomes. Even with the highest resolution karyotype, the average chromosome band equals about 2×10^6 bp. These measurements emphasize the vastly greater precision of molecular analysis in detecting gene deletions (40,000 bp) or codon deletions as in the F_{508} mutation (i.e., the deletion of a phenylalanine codon that is common in cystic fibrosis).

411–412. The answers are: 411-A, 412-C. *(Gelehrter, pp 82–84, 290. Thompson, 5/e, pp 110, 176–177.)* The polymerase chain reaction (PCR) is a technique in which thermal cycling is used to amplify small segments of DNA rapidly. This technique is useful for the amplification of samples of DNA as small as those contained in a single haploid cell (e.g., a human sperm). Pulsed-field gel electrophoresis is a technique in which segments of DNA as large as 10 million bp may be reliably separated. By combining this technique with restriction enzymes that cut only rarely, fragments of DNA in the range of 1 million base pairs are generated, and physical maps may be created.

413–414. The answers are: 413-A, 414-C. *(Gelehrter, pp 90–93. Thompson, 5/e, pp 48–51.)* The promoter region of DNA is located in the 5′ region of the gene that determines the site of initiation of transcription; it is also known as the cap site. The promoter may also help regulate the quantity and the tissue specificity of messenger RNA (mRNA).

The polyadenylation site is located at the 3′ end of mRNA. It is the location at which approximately 200 adenosine residues (poly-A tail) is added. This poly-A tail assists in the transport of the mRNA out of the nucleus and adds to its stability. Cryptic splice sites are sequences of DNA that are similar to the normal (consensus) splice sites. When the consensus splice site is mutated, the cryptic splice site may be used.

415–417. The answers are: 415-B, 416-C, 417-E. *(Gelehrter, pp 17–18. Thompson, 5/e, pp 33–36.)* DNA is "packaged" via an efficient method of coiling; that is, it is wound around proteins called histones, which are rich in basic amino acids. Together these condensed packages of DNA and proteins are called chromatin. Heterochromatin is chromatin that contains repetitive DNA and that stains darkly with trypsin and Giemsa. The centromere, also known as the primary constriction, is a region of heterochromatin by which sister chromatids are held together. Spindle fibers attach at the centromere to a structure called the kinetochore.

418–420. The answers are: 418-D, 419-B, 420-A. *(Gelehrter, pp 11–12. Thompson, 5/e, pp 31–33.)* DNA is composed of a backbone of deoxyribose, a sugar, each with an associated phosphate, which are attached by 5'-3' phosphodiester bonds. Attached to each sugar is one of four nitrogen-containing bases. Two of the bases are purines (adenine and guanine) and two are pyrimidines (thymine and cytosine). Each unit composed of a sugar, phosphate, and base is known as a nucleotide. Two complimentary strands of DNA are attached via hydrogen bonds, which form between adenine and thymine or between guanine and cytosine. In RNA, the sugar ribose replaces deoxyribose.

421–423. The answers are: 421-B, 422-A, 423-D. *(Gelehrter, pp 69–121. Thompson, 5/e, pp 97–114.)* Exons are the coding portions of genes and consist of trinucleotide codons that guide the placement of specific amino acids into protein. Introns are the noncoding portions of genes that may function in evolution to provide "shuffling" of exons to produce new proteins. The primary RNA transcript contains both exons and introns, but the latter are removed by RNA splicing. The 5' (upstream) and 3' (downstream) untranslated RNA regions remain in the mature RNA and are thought to regulate RNA transport or translation. A poly(A) tail is added to the primary transcript after transcription, which facilitates transport and processing from the nucleus. The discovery of introns complicated Mendel's idea of the gene as the smallest hereditary unit; a modern definition might be the colinear sequence of exons, introns, and adjacent regulatory sequences that accomplish protein expression. Using these principles, one can determine the size of the stimulin gene. It contains a coding region of 300 bp (100 amino acids $\times$ 3 bp per amino acid) plus 100 bp in the intron, plus 70 + 30 = 100 bp in the untranslated regions (total = 500 bp). The mature RNA contains the same number of bp except for the 100 bp in the intron (500 − 100 = 400 bp). Transcription begins at the start of the 5' untranslated region (70 bp) and the splice site occurs 30 bp (10 $\times$ 3) into the coding region at the beginning of the intron (70 + 30 = 100 bp).

424–426. The answers are: 424-B, 425-A, 426-D. *(Gelehrter, pp 9–17. Thompson, 5/e, pp 40–41.)* DNA is duplicated in a process called replication. The annealing of two complementary strands of DNA is called hybridization. Double-stranded DNA is transcribed into single-stranded messenger RNA (mRNA), which can then be translated with the help of amino acid–specific transfer RNAs (tRNAs) into polypeptide chains.

427–429. The answers are: 427-B, 428-D, 429-A. *(Gelehrter, pp 193–228. Thompson, 5/e, pp 115–142.)* The analysis in the figure that accompanies the question demonstrates the greater power and sensitivity of variable numbers of tandem repeats (VNTRs) for linkage studies. Regions with variable numbers of CA (dinucleotide) repeats are widely dispersed in the genome, so that VNTRs are now available for genetic linkage and mapping of most disease loci. The polymerase chain reaction (PCR) amplification, using primers that bracket the variable region, yield discrete bands that reflect the distance between primers, including the number of dinucleotide repeats (*bottom of figure*). Because the resulting alleles differ in size by only a few nucleotides, high-resolution gels must be used for separation of the amplified fragments. Alleles can be read directly from the gel, and their diversity allows easy tracking of the nail-patella allele based on linkage to VNTR allele 1.

430–432. The answers are: 430-E, 431-B, 432-D. *(Gelehrter, pp 193–228. Thompson, 5/e, pp 115–142.)* Individual II-3 has alleles 1 and 4 (genotype 1,4) based on the DNA analysis shown in the figure that accompanies the previous question. Her husband has genotype 2,4 with possible fetal genotypes 1,2 (affected); 1,4 (affected); 2,4 (unaffected); and 4,4 (unaffected). Individual II-5 also has genotype 1,4 as deduced from DNA analysis, so that mating with a man of genotype 1,5 should not yield a fetus of genotype 1,2. Uniparental disomy would also not explain this fetal genotype, leaving nonpaternity as the most likely possibility. This is the reason that full consent for DNA analysis should include mention that results will indicate nonpaternity if present. Individual III-3 has alleles 1 and 5, so that a fetus with genotype 2,5 inherited the maternal variable number of tandem repeats (VNTRs) allele that is not linked to the nail-patella syndrome.

433–435. The answers are: 433-D, 434-B, 435-A. *(Gelehrter, pp 21–22. Thompson, 5/e, pp 131–138.)* A mutation is a permanent change in DNA. Many different types of mutations are possible. The most common types of mutations are point mutations in which one nucleotide is simply substituted for another. These may be *missense mutations,* resulting in the substitution of one amino acid residue for another, *nonsense mutations,* resulting in premature stop signals, or *silent mutations* where the substitution does not alter the amino acid sequence. Occasionally, point mutations may alter splice sites or regulatory elements. Deletions may be as small as a single nucleotide or very large, eliminating whole genes or more. When deletions eliminate nucleotides in multiples of three (the length of individual codons), amino acid residues are lost. However, when deletions involve other numbers of nucleotides, the reading frame of the gene may be altered. Such mutations, often called frameshift mutations, change all subsequent amino acids and may result in premature stops.

436–437. The answers are: 436-C, 437-E. *(Gelehrter, pp 71–78. Thompson, 5/e, pp 97–114.)* Nucleic acid hybridization involves the reassociation of DNA-DNA, DNA-RNA, or RNA-RNA complementary strands under controlled conditions. Inclusion of a radioactive or chemically labeled DNA or RNA segment (probe) allows quantitation of hybridization at the end of the reaction. Oligonucleotides are short (15 to 50 base pairs), artificially synthesized DNA or RNA segments that may be employed as primers to initiate DNA sequencing or polymerase chain reactions (PCRs). The short length may also be used to advantage in stringent hybridization reactions to discriminate among alleles differing by a single base pair [allele-specific oligonucleotides (ASOs)]. Recombinant DNA molecules containing specific DNA sequences are referred to as clones. They may be inserted into vectors, which then replicate, creating large quantities of the DNA fragment of interest. Common cloning vectors include plasmids, cosmids, and bacteriophages.

438–439. The answers are: 438-D, 439-E. *(Gelehrter, pp 91–92. Thompson, 5/e, pp 50, 385.)* *Homeobox genes* are important in developmental control. In *Drosophila,* mutations in these genes may alter the development of the different body segments. *Housekeeping genes* provide basic functions and are constitutively expressed in all tissues. The promoters of these genes are frequently unusual in that they do not contain CAT and TATA boxes that help regulate transcription. These promoters frequently contain relatively large amounts of cytosine and guanine and may be located in the regions of the genome referred to as CG or CpG islands.

    Structural genes code for RNA and protein products. *Oncogenes* act in a dominant fashion to promote cell growth and may lead to neoplastic transformation. *Tumor suppressor genes* block abnormal growth. Recessive mutations in these genes may also lead to neoplastic transformation.

440–441. The answers are: 440-B, 441-C. *(Gelehrter, pp 69–94. Thompson, 5/e, pp 40–51.)* In general, genes contain coding sequences, or exons, which are interrupted by intervening sequences, or introns. These intronic sequences are removed during the processing of RNA. Intergenic DNA is located between the genes and is untranscribed. Pseudogenes closely resemble genes but are nonfunctional.

442–444. The answers are: 442-C, 443-E, 444-D. *(Gelehrter, pp 193–228. Thompson, 5/e, pp 115–142.)* The analysis of the figure that accompanies the question is typical of diseases caused by instability of trinucleotide repeats. This is a growing category of disease that includes fragile X syndrome, Huntington's chorea, myotonic dystrophy, and others. Once the region of triplet repeat instability is cloned, polymerase chain reaction (PCR) analysis, using primers bracketing the triplet repeats, can discriminate among normal individuals (e.g., individual II-4), individuals with "premutations" that have a high risk for amplification during meiosis (e.g., individual I-1), and full mutations associated with disease symptoms (e.g., individuals II-2 and II-3). Although it is unusual for carriers of X-linked recessive disorders to be symptomatic, 50 percent of females with sufficient amplification of trinucleotide repeats adjacent to the fragile X mental retardation (FMR-1) gene have mental retardation.

445–447. The answers are: 445-E, 446-A, 447-C. *(Gelehrter, pp 193–228. Thompson, 5/e, pp 115–142.)* Triplet repeat diseases are characterized by dramatic instability of trinucleotide repeats once they reach an intermediate number. For fragile X syndrome, this "premutation" ranges between 52 and 230 repeats and is most likely to amplify into the symptomatic range during female meiosis. Fragile X males and symptomatic female carriers with large numbers of trinucleotide repeats show instability during embryogenesis with various tissues having different repeat numbers. This somatic mosaicism for repeat numbers produces the smear of differently sized DNA fragments diagrammed for individuals II-2 and II-3 in the figure that accompanies the previous question. Individuals with normal numbers of trinucleotide repeats have virtually no risk of having a child with fragile X syndrome. Males with "premutations" of 52 to 230 repeats also have a minimal risk of having symptomatic carrier daughters, but these daughters have a risk for affected sons because of amplification during female meiosis.

448–451. The answers are: 448-F, 449-A, 450-F, 451-E. *(Gelehrter, pp 21–22, 76–88. Thompson, 5/e, pp 106–108, 131–140.)* Molecular genetic techniques allow the analysis of gene structure and function. However, results of such testing cannot be evaluated in isolation. Point mutations in noncoding regions may alter sites for restriction endonuclease cleavage and, therefore, give abnormal patterns on Southern blotting, without altering the function of the gene itself. Conversely, missense mutations, which cause the substitution of one amino acid for another, may significantly alter the function of the resultant protein without altering the electrophoretic pattern seen on Southern blotting. In this case, Northern blot results would most likely also be normal. Single-base changes may also result in nonsense mutations. These mutations are likely to result in abnormal messenger RNA (mRNA) patterns and abnormal, truncated, and highly unstable proteins. Deletions of the entire gene will obviously result in the absence of all mRNA and no enzymatic activity.

452–454. The answers are: 452-D, 453-B, 454-E. *(Gelehrter, pp 21–22. Thompson, 5/e, pp 115–144.)* The genetic code employs sets of three bases,

known as codons, to specify the 20 different amino acids. Since more combinations of bases (64 three-base combinations) are possible than the number of
amino acids, each amino acid may be coded for by more than one combination. Additionally, some codons represent a "stop" or chain termination signal. Mutations alter the meaning of the DNA sequence, just as typographical
errors alter the meaning of a sentence. Point mutations, which alter a single
base, may result either in a substitution of one amino acid for another or, if the
change results in a stop codon, may prematurely end the amino acid chain.
The codon for methionine initiates the reading of the DNA sequence and
establishes the reading frame. In-frame deletions cause the loss of single
amino acids. However, out-of-frame deletions alter the meaning or amino
acid sequence of the remainder of the protein. Since several different codons
may code for the same amino acids, some base substitutions, known also as
silent mutations, may occur, which do not change the amino acid sequence
at all.

Integrated Cases and Ethics

DIRECTIONS: Each question below contains four or five suggested responses. Select the **one best** response to each question. For these integrated cases, negatively and positively phrased questions are not separated.

Questions 455–459

455. A 6-year-old girl is referred to a physician for evaluation. She is known to have mild mental retardation and a ventricular septal defect (VSD). The physician asks the parents for all the following information EXCEPT

(A) family history of learning problems
(B) folate prior to and during pregnancy
(C) medications or drugs taken during pregnancy
(D) early developmental milestones
(E) parental consanguinity

456. On physical examination, the patient is noted to have some facial dysmorphism, including a long face, a prominent nose, and flattening in the malar region. In addition, the patient's speech has an unusual quality. Which description best explains the patient's condition?

A) Sequence
B) Syndrome
C) Disruption
D) Deformation
E) Single birth defect

457. A standard karyotypic analysis is ordered for this patient, the results of which are normal. A colleague recommends performing fluorescent in situ hybridization (FISH) analysis on the patient's chromosomes, using probes for chromosome 22. Only one signal is seen for each chromosomal spread. Which of the following statements regarding these analyses is true?

(A) The initial karyotype results are inconsistent with the FISH results
(B) This is a normal result
(C) A small deletion is present on one of the patient's number 22 chromosomes
(D) FISH is only helpful when the initial karyotype results are abnormal
(E) The chromosome with the positive signal is paternal in origin

458. Based on these test results, the physician makes a diagnosis of velo-cardiofacial syndrome, a condition associated with a deletion on chromosome 22. A multispecialty approach to this patient would include all of the following professionals EXCEPT a

(A) cardiologist
(B) pediatrician
(C) speech therapist
(D) physical therapist
(E) family therapist

459. Fluorescent in situ hybridization (FISH) analysis is useful in all the following situations EXCEPT

(A) syndrome identification
(B) determination of sex in cases of ambiguous genitalia
(C) determination of uniparental disomy
(D) rapid diagnosis of trisomies
(E) identification of submicroscopic deletions

Questions 460–470

A child is referred for evaluation of developmental delay and unusual behavior. On examination, the physician notes loose joints, large ears, prominent jaw, and large testes for age.

460. This child's condition is most likely to be a

(A) sequence
(B) syndrome
(C) disruption
(D) single birth defect
(E) deformation

461. A karyotype should be considered for the child because

(A) most children with mental retardation have chromosomal aberrations
(B) mental retardation (developmental delay) and multiple major or minor anomalies are hallmarks of chromosomal disease
(C) the patient has several characteristics of Down syndrome
(D) Klinefelter syndrome (47,XXY) is associated with megalotestes

462. The karyotype obtained from this child with developmental delay was first read as normal. Another physician, suspicious of a particular disease, ordered a second karyotype that is performed in a special cell medium and obtained the result 46,XY,fra(X). The required cell medium was

(A) high calcium medium
(B) low calcium medium
(C) low phosphate medium
(D) low folic acid medium
(E) high folic acid medium

463. A family history was obtained for this child with developmental delay. The child's mother had learning disabilities and only finished the ninth grade. Two maternal uncles had more severe mental retardation and required special education. The full pedigree is shown in the figure below, with filled symbols representing severe mental retardation and hatched symbols representing learning disabilities. The most likely inheritance pattern is

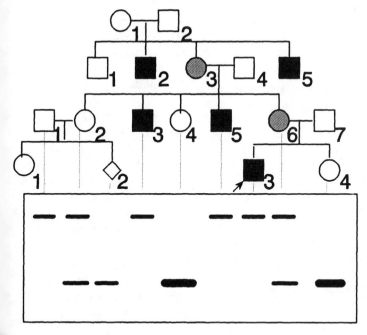

A) autosomal recessive
B) autosomal dominant
C) X-linked recessive
D) mitochondrial

464. The diagnosis is fragile X syndrome. Given the pedigree illustrated, what is the risk that individual III-6 will have a severely affected male in a future pregnancy?

(A) 100 percent
(B) 50 percent
(C) 25 percent
(D) 12.5 percent
(E) Virtually 0

465. Ignoring the Southern blot below the pedigree, what is the risk that individual III-4 will have a severely affected male?

(A) 100 percent
(B) 50 percent
(C) 25 percent
(D) 12.5 percent
(E) Virtually 0

466. What is the risk that individual IV-3 will have a severely affected male?

(A) 100 percent
(B) 50 percent
(C) 25 percent
(D) 12.5 percent
(E) Virtually 0

467. To determine the risk for transmitting fragile X syndrome, karyotyping would be useful for which individuals in the illustrated pedigree?

(A) III-2, III-4, IV-1, IV-4
(B) III-2, III-4
(C) III-2, III-4, III-6
(D) III-2, III-4, III-6, IV-1, IV-4
(E) IV-1, IV-3, IV-4

468. Because older female carriers of fragile X syndrome often do not exhibit the fragile site, alternative diagnostic testing is needed to determine their carrier status. The hypothetical Southern blot shown under the illustrated pedigree displays the DNA restriction fragments visualized with the probe DXS548 corresponding to individuals from the pedigree. DXS548 is a single-copy polymorphic locus that has been mapped to within 1 megabase of the fra(X) site. Based on these data, what is the risk that individual III-2 will have a son with the fragile X syndrome?

(A) 100 percent
(B) 50 percent
(C) 25 percent
(D) 12.5 percent
(E) Virtually 0

469. Individual III-2 of the pedigree and blot illustrated has requested prenatal diagnosis for her 16-week pregnancy. A fetal karyotype did not show the fragile X marker, and the DNA analysis is shown in the figure under individual IV-2. Based on these results, the most likely prenatal diagnosis and its accuracy are

(A) normal female, 95 percent
(B) carrier female, 95 percent
(C) unaffected male, 99 percent
(D) affected male, 99 percent

470. Suppose that individual III-2 had become estranged from her family and that her relatives refused to give permission for release of their positive fragile X testing results. Which of the following ethical principles and possible outcomes would the family physician confront if he or she notified individual III-2 of her risks?

(A) Informed consent, medical commendation
(B) Informed consent, legal liability
(C) Patient confidentiality, medical commendation
(D) Patient confidentiality, legal liability
(E) None of the above

(end of group questions)

471. In 1991, it was discovered that the fragile X syndrome was caused by a mutation in the fragile X mental retardation-1 (FMR1) gene. An area of CGG trinucleotide repeats just upstream of the coding area was found to be variable in size. All the following statements regarding the FMR1 gene are true EXCEPT

(A) the length of this region is variable in normal individuals
(B) "premutations" may expand to full mutations in future generations
(C) individuals with premutations are likely to have mental retardation
(D) offspring of male carriers inherit a premutation
(E) offspring of female carriers may inherit a premutation or a full mutation

---

Questions 472–476

472. A child is referred for evaluation because of low muscle tone and developmental delay. Shortly after delivery the child was a poor feeder and had to be fed by tube. In the second year, the child began to eat voraciously and became obese. He also had a slightly unusual face with almond-shaped eyes and downturned corners of the mouth. The hands, feet, and penis were small, and the scrotum was poorly formed. The diagnostic category and laboratory test to be considered for this child are

(A) sequence, serum testosterone
(B) single birth defect, serum testosterone
(C) deformation, karyotype
(D) syndrome, karyotype
(E) disruption, karyotype

473. A karyotype was performed on the obese child and was entirely normal. Because his physician suspected a disorder known as Prader-Willi syndrome, Southern blotting was performed to determine the origin of the patient's number 15 chromosomes. In part A of the figure below, a hypothetical Southern blot with DNA probe D15S8 defines which of four restriction fragment length polymorphisms (RFLPs) are present in DNA from mother (M), child (C), and father (F). Based on the D15S8 locus, what is the origin of the child's two number 15 chromosomes?

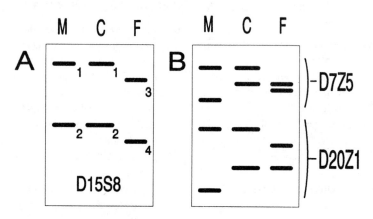

(A) One from the mother, one from the father
(B) Both from the father
(C) Both from the mother
(D) Results cannot be interpreted

474. Because part A of the figure demonstrates that the child is missing both paternal chromosome 15 alleles, nonpaternity would be a more plausible explanation than uniparental disomy. The hypothetical Southern blot shown in part B illustrates a DNA "fingerprinting" analysis to examine paternity, where maternal (M), child (C), and paternal (F) DNA samples have been restricted, blotted, and hybridized simultaneously to the probes D7Z5 and D20Z1. The distributions of restriction fragment alleles suggests

(A) the child is adopted
(B) false maternity (i.e., baby switched in the nursery)
(C) false paternity
(D) correct maternity and paternity
(E) None of the above

475. As discussed in the previous question, the DNA analyses in the figure have the potential to demonstrate nonpaternity. If the physician ordering these analyses did not discuss this possibility with the mother, he or she would be in violation of

(A) patient confidentiality
(B) patient rights
(C) informed consent
(D) standards of care
(E) malpractice guidelines

476. Given that the analysis in part B of the figure excludes nonpaternity, the chromosome 15 restriction fragment alleles revealed in part A become predictive of particular chromosomal anomalies. The presence of restriction fragment alleles 1 and 2 detected in the child as represented in part A implies

(A) uniparental disomy (maternal isodisomy 15)
(B) uniparental disomy (maternal heterodisomy 15)
(C) uniparental disomy (maternal isodisomy 15) or monosomy 15
(D) trisomy 15 due to maternal nondisjunction
(E) trisomy 15 due to paternal nondisjunction

(end of group questions)

Questions 477–480

477. The genesis of Prader-Willi syndrome by inheritance of two normal chromosomes from a single parent is an example of

(A) germinal mosaicism
(B) genomic imprinting
(C) chromosome deletion
(D) chromosome rearrangement
(E) anticipation

478. A child has severe epilepsy with fits of laughing, developmental delay, short stature, and autistic behavior. Her appetite is normal. The family history revealed three normal siblings, normal parents, no consanguinity, and two normal aunts and uncles on each side of the family. The family history rules out

(A) autosomal recessive disease
(B) autosomal dominant disease
(C) X-linked dominant disease
(D) chromosomal disease
(E) multigenerational disease

479. The child in the previous question has characteristic manifestations of a condition known as the *Angelman syndrome*. Because of the syndromic nature of the disorder and the developmental delay, a karyotype is performed and yields the chromosomes 15 shown below. The partial karyotype reveals

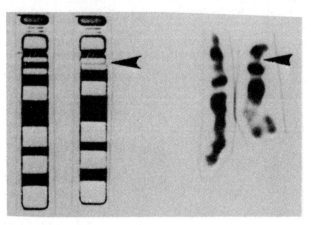

(A) interstitial deletion of 15q
(B) interstitial deletion of 15p
(C) pericentric inversion of 15
(D) paracentric inversion of 15
(E) none of the above

480. A Southern blot analysis is performed on the patient discussed in the previous two questions using the probe D15S8. Assume that the parental restriction fragment alleles were the same as those in the figure at question 473. What conclusion could be drawn if the child's analysis revealed the presence of only allele 3?

(A) Paternal heterodisomy 15
(B) Biparental contribution of chromosomes 15, D15S8 locus within deleted region, deletion occurred on paternal 15
(C) Biparental contribution of chromosomes 15, D15S8 locus within deleted region, deletion occurred on maternal 15
(D) Biparental contribution of chromosomes 15, D15S8 locus not within deleted region
(E) None of above

(end of group questions)

481. Questions 472 through 480 illustrated that a patient with deletion of the maternal 15q13q15 region may have Angelman syndrome and a patient with maternal heterodisomy for chromosome 15 may have Prader-Willi syndrome. These observations may be reconciled because

(A) lack of a paternally derived 15q13q15 region produces Angelman syndrome, and lack of a maternally derived 15q13q15 region produces Prader-Willi syndrome
(B) lack of a maternally derived 15q13q15 region produces Angelman syndrome, and lack of a paternally derived 15q13q15 region produces Prader-Willi syndrome
(C) deletion of 15q13q15 produces Angelman syndrome, while uniparental disomy 15 produces Prader-Willi syndrome
(D) deletion of 15q13q15 produces Prader-Willi syndrome, while uniparental disomy 15 produces Angelman syndrome

Questions 482–485

A newborn presents with ambiguous genitalia as seen in the figure below. The photograph shows an enlarged clitoris or small phallus with labial fusion or hypoplastic scrotum.

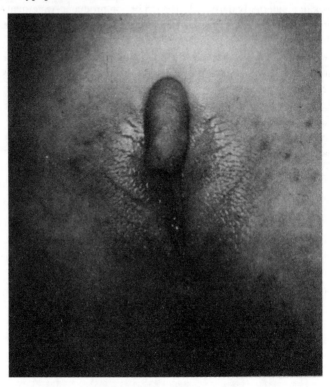

482. This child's sex is most reliably established by

(A) buccal smear to determine if there are one or two Barr bodies
(B) buccal smear to determine if there is one Barr body or none
(C) peripheral blood karyotype
(D) bone marrow karyotype
(E) polymerase chain reaction (PCR), using primers specific for the long arm of the Y chromosome

483. The dot-blot shown below examines the proband's DNA after polymerase chain reaction (PCR) amplification and hybridization with DNA probes from the X and Y chromosome. In this case, the Y chromosome probe is from the SRY region of Yp that has recently been characterized as the male-determining region. DNA from control male and female patients is also applied to the dot-blot. Based on the dot-blot results, which of the following conclusions can be reached?

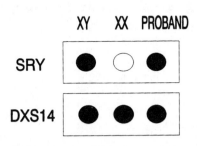

(A) The proband is a genetic male
(B) The proband is a genetic female
(C) The proband is male
(D) The proband is female
(E) None of the above

484. Based on the photograph and dot-blot analysis, the anomaly illustrated is

(A) female pseudohermaphroditism
(B) male pseudohermaphroditism
(C) true hermaphroditism
(D) an XY female
(E) an XX male

485. The physician received the karyotype result on the proband and it was 46,XY. The most likely diagnosis was local failure of the external genitalia to respond to testosterone, and this was supported by studies excluding defects of pituitary-adrenal function and of the internal genitalia. The physician chose not to tell the parents that their child was actually a genetic male but emphasized that she was a female who should return for management at puberty because of the risk of sexual and reproductive problems. From the ethical perspective, this action would fall under the category of

(A) patient confidentiality
(B) nondisclosure
(C) informed consent
(D) failure to provide ongoing care
(E) discrimination

(end of group questions)

Questions 486–492

An infant presents at day 10 of life with poor feeding, vomiting, and lethargy.

486. Which of the following diagnoses could you immediately eliminate?

(A) Syndrome
(B) Sepsis
(C) Cardiomyopathy
(D) Central nervous system (CNS) catastrophy
(E) Inborn error of metabolism

487. Further history reveals that the infant was the full-term product of a normal pregnancy and delivery. He did well in the first 48 hours of life and was discharged home with his mother. The infant then developed progressive lethargy, anorexia, and vomiting over the next week. In evaluating the possibility of an inborn error of metabolism, which of the following is an unimportant piece of information?

(A) Family history of neonatal deaths
(B) Family history of consanguinity
(C) Infant's feeding history
(D) Any unusual odors
(E) Parental karyotypes

488. Laboratory tests reveal a low white blood cell count, metabolic acidosis, increased anion gap, and mild hyperammonemia. Measurement of plasma amino acids reveals elevated levels of glycine, and measurement of urinary organic acids reveals increased amounts of propionic acid and methyl citrate. A diagnosis of propionic acidemia is made. The family history reveals that the parents are first cousins. This disorder is likely to be

(A) autosomal dominant
(B) autosomal recessive
(C) X-linked dominant
(D) X-linked recessive
(E) multifactorial

489. Propionic acidemia is caused by a deficiency of propionyl-CoA carboxylase (PCC), as shown in the following reaction:

Valine
Odd-chain fatty acids   PCC
Methionine   →   propionyl-   ↛   methylmalonyl-CoA
Isoleucine   CoA
Threonine   ↓
                                 propionic acid
                                 methyl citrate

In the treatment of this disorder, which of the following would be contraindicated?

(A) Antibiotics
(B) A diet high in valine, isoleucine, and methionine
(C) Caloric supplementation
(D) Aggressive fluid and electrolyte management
(E) Hemodialysis

490. Biotin is a cofactor in the reaction catalyzed by propionyl–coenzyme A (CoA) carboxylase (PCC) as well as several other carboxylases. In holocarboxylase synthase deficiency, none of these carboxylases can be made. A similar picture may be seen in biotinidase deficiency, a disorder of biotin metabolism. These disorders constitute an example of

(A) allelic heterogeneity
(B) genetic heterogeneity
(C) variable expressivity
(D) incomplete penetrance
(E) dosage compensation

491. The parents of the proband in this family return to the physician's office 2 years later. The mother of the proband is pregnant. The risk that the fetus is affected with propionic acidemia is

(A) 2/3
(B) 1/2
(C) 1/4
(D) 1/8
(E) virtually 0

492. DNA analysis is performed on the family. Results are shown in the figure below. The risk that the fetus is affected with propionic acidemia is now

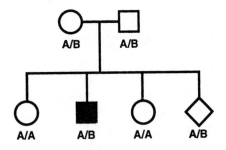

(A) virtually 100 percent
(B) 2/3
(C) 1/2
(D) 1/4
(E) virtually 0

(end of group questions)

Questions 493–495

A 1-year-old boy (proband) seemed normal at birth but developed a large liver, cloudy cornea and skeletal anomalies. His mental development was also delayed. His clinical and developmental course are very reminiscent of two older sisters who have been diagnosed with Hurler syndrome, a metabolic storage disease in which mucopolysaccharides accumulate in many tissues. The remainder of the family history is unremarkable except that the parents are first cousins.

493. What is the risk of the parents of the proband having another child with Hurler syndrome?

  (A) 1/2
  (B) 1/4
  (C) 3/4
  (D) 1/12
  (E) 1/24

494. What is the risk of the normal sibling and the proband having a child with Hurler syndrome if she marries a first cousin on her mother's side of the family?

  (A) 1/2
  (B) 1/4
  (C) 3/4
  (D) 1/12
  (E) 1/24

495. What is the risk of a normal sibling of the proband having a child with Hurler syndrome if she marries an unrelated individual, given that the incidence of Hurler syndrome is 1/10,000?

  (A) 1/48
  (B) 1/96
  (C) 1/200
  (D) 1/300
  (E) 1/600

(end of group questions)

---

496. In addition to the Hurler syndrome, at least six other mucopolysaccharidoses have been identified. Many have a similar phenotype, which includes coarse facial features, skeletal disease, and variable intellectual retardation. The finding that coculture of fibroblasts from patients in different disease groups corrected the mucopolysaccharide degradation defect was instrumental in the delineation of these diseases. The name for this phenomenon (and its genetic implication) is

(A) complementation (allelic heterogeneity)
(B) complementation (genetic heterogeneity)
(C) somatic cell hybridization (allelic heterogeneity)
(D) somatic cell hybridization (genetic heterogeneity)

497. Hurler syndrome is caused by a deficiency of the enzyme L-iduronidase. It was demonstrated by Neufeld that exogenous L-iduronidase could be taken up by deficient cells via a targeting signal that directed the enzyme to its normal lysosomal location. All of the therapeutic strategies below might be considered for affected children EXCEPT

(A) germ-line gene therapy
(B) heterologous bone marrow transplant to provide a source of enzyme
(C) infection with a disabled adenovirus vector that carries the L-iduronidase gene
(D) injection with L-iduronidase purified from human liver
(E) autologous bone marrow transplant after transfection with a virus carrying the L-iduronidase gene

498. The parents of the 1-year-old boy in questions 493–495 decided to pursue bone marrow transplantation for their youngest child. Because gene therapy was not yet available, they decided to consider the three normal siblings as donors. Preliminary testing of these normal siblings was performed to assess their carrier status and their human leukocyte antigen (HLA) locus compatibility with the affected brother. What is the chance that one of the three siblings will be homozygous normal (i.e., have a good supply of enzyme) and HLA compatible?

(A) 1/2
(B) 1/3
(C) 1/4
(D) 1/6
(E) 1/12

499. A sibling donor was found for the patient, and the physician wrote to the patient's insurance company explaining the diagnosis of Hurler syndrome and the reasons for bone marrow transplant. Not only did the insurance company refuse payment for transplantation, they also discontinued coverage for the family based on anticipated medical expenses. From the ethical perspective, these events would fall under which of the following categories?

(A) Patient confidentiality
(B) Nondisclosure
(C) Informed consent
(D) Failure to provide ongoing care
(E) Discrimination

500. Hurler syndrome results from a deficiency of α-L-iduronidase, an enzyme that catalyzes degradation of mucopolysaccharides in lysosomes. This enzyme is present in all embryonic tissues. Prenatal diagnosis of the couple's next pregnancy could be theoretically accomplished by all the following EXCEPT

(A) chorionic villi sampling (CVS)
(B) percutaneous umbilical blood sampling
(C) amniocentesis
(D) maternal serum α-fetoprotein (MSAFP)

Integrated Cases and Ethics

Answers

455. The answer is B. *(Gelehrter, pp 255–262. Thompson, 5/e, pp 391–394.)* Taking a family history is a crucial ingredient in making the diagnosis of a genetic disease. It should be relevant to the clinical details of the case, and, if possible, should include information relating to multiple generations, ethnic and racial background, and a history of consanguinity. Evaluation of any child should always include a developmental history. Teratogen exposure is also important in assessing any problem that appears congenital. Recently, folate deficiency in the periconceptional period has been associated with neural tube defects.

456. The answer is B. *(Thompson, 5/e, pp 391–392.)* The child described in the question has multiple independent anomalies that are characteristic of a syndrome. Although they are likely to be causally related, they do not appear to be sequential. These problems do not appear to be caused by the breakdown of an originally normal developmental process as in a disruption, nor do they appear to be related to a nondisruptive mechanical force as in a deformation.

457. The answer is C. *(Isselbacher, 13/e, pp 373–374.)* Fluorescent in situ hybridization (FISH) analysis is a technique in which molecular probes that are specific for individual chromosomes or chromosomal regions are used to identify these regions. FISH probes frequently identify chromosomal regions that are submicroscopic and, therefore, may be useful when standard karyotypic analysis is normal. In this case, the fact that only one signal is present despite the fact that there are two number 22 chromosomes, indicates that a submicroscopic deletion has occurred. The parental chromosome of origin cannot be determined using this technique unless that parent also carries a similar deletion and his or her chromosomes are evaluated.

458. The answer is D. *(Gelehrter, pp 255–262. Thompson, 5/e, pp 395–404.)* Genetics is not an organ system–directed subspecialty, such as cardiology or nephrology. Therefore, patients with genetic diseases frequently need multiple subspecialists to help care for their multiple problems. It is crucial to understand the enormous physical, emotional, and financial burden that these disorders place not only on the patient but on the family as well. Family counseling and individual counseling are important aspects of the care of these patients. It is important to include the primary care physicians as they frequently serve as coordinators of care.

459. The answer is C. *(Isselbacher, 13/e, pp 373–374. Thompson, 5/e, p 175.)* The availability of specific molecular probes allows the use of fluorescent in situ hybridization (FISH) analysis for the evaluation of specific chromosomal regions known to be associated with specific genetic syndromes. Probes specific for the X and Y chromosomes are used in determining sex in cases of ambiguous genitalia. The identification of three signals for specific chromosomes allows for the diagnosis of trisomies much more rapidly than standard karyotypic analysis. Submicroscopic deletions can be detected using FISH probes. Because the parental chromosome of origin cannot be determined with this technique, uniparental disomy cannot be detected.

460. The answer is B. *(Thompson, 5/e, p 391.)* A pattern of major or minor anomalies is known as a *syndrome.* The child's minor abnormalities plus developmental delay are strongly suggestive of a syndrome. It is important to distinguish syndromes from sequences (i.e., multiple consequences produced by a single embryologic error) or isolated birth defects (i.e., disruptions, deformations, and malformations) since the latter categories usually have an optimistic prognosis with minimum recurrence risk.

461. The answer is B. *(Gelehrter, pp 171–176.)* Mental retardation of unknown cause, particularly when accompanied by multiple major or minor anomalies, is an indication for karyotyping. The child's facial appearance and minor anomalies are atypical of Down syndrome. Males with Klinefelter syndrome have small rather than large testes.

462. The answer is D. *(Gelehrter, pp 185–187. Thompson, 5/e, pp 81–82.)* The fra(X) notation indicates a discontinuity near the tip of the X long arm. Cytogenetic visualization of this fragile site requires lymphocyte culture in low folic acid medium before metaphase arrest. Originally noticed by chance, the 46,XY,fra(X) karyotype is now associated with a fragile X syndrome of mental retardation, loose joints, characteristic facies, and megalotestes.

463. The answer is C. *(Gelehrter, pp 39–45. Thompson, 5/e, pp 75–80.)* The pedigree that accompanies the question demonstrates oblique transmission with severely affected males and normal or mildly affected females. X-linked recessive inheritance is most likely, although X-linked dominant inheritance with variable, milder expression in females is also possible. The lack of phenotypic findings in individual I-1 argues against X-linked dominant inheritance since her two affected sons indicate that she has the abnormal allele.

464. The answer is C. *(Gelehrter, pp 39–45. Thompson, 5/e, pp 75–80.)* Individual III-6 is an obligate carrier because of her affected son. She has a 1/2 chance for a son and a 1/2 chance for the son to have the fragile X syndrome, which results in a $1/2 \times 1/2 = 1/4$ overall risk.

465. The answer is D. *(Gelehrter, pp 39–45. Thompson, 5/e, pp 75–80.)* Individual III-4 has a 1/2 chance to be a carrier and a 1/4 chance to have an affected son if she is a carrier. This results in a $1/2 \times 1/4 = 1/8$ overall risk.

466. The answer is E. *(Gelehrter, pp 39–45. Thompson, 5/e, pp 75–80.)* Affected males, such as individual IV-3, cannot transmit their abnormal X chromosome allele to sons.

467. The answer is A. *(Gelehrter, pp 185–187. Thompson, 5/e, pp 81–82.)* Females may transmit abnormal X chromosomal alleles but be unaffected themselves because of the normal X chromosomal allele. Females at risk to be carriers of X-linked recessive diseases, thus, need counseling and detection of their carrier status where possible. Some female carriers of the fragile X chromosome show the fragile X site by karyotyping under appropriate culture conditions.

468. The answer is C. *(Gelehrter, pp 193–207. Thompson, 5/e, pp 420–423.)* The restriction fragment allele of lower molecular weight (nearer the bottom of the hypothetical autoradiogram in the figure) is linked to the normal X chromosome allele. Individual III-2 is, thus, definitely a carrier. Phase (which new restriction fragment length polymorphism [RFLP] allele segregates with the disease allele) is easily established in X-linked disorders by noting the restriction fragment present in affected males.

469. The answer is C. *(Gelehrter, pp 193–207. Thompson, 5/e, pp 420–423.)* The fetus has received the lower molecular weight restriction fragment allele from his mother and is at minimal risk to have fragile X syndrome. The fetus must be male since he has received neither paternal X chromosome allele. Accuracy of the diagnosis depends on the chance of recombination between the restriction fragment and fragile X loci. The distance between these loci is indicated as <1 megabase in the previous question. This distance is approximately equivalent to 1 centimorgan (cM) or a 1 percent chance of recombination.

470. The answer is D. *(Thompson, 5/e, p 395.)* Genetic counseling, like other medical practice, entails privileged communication between patient and physician. All information regarding the patient is confidential and cannot be shared with any institution or individual without the patient's written permission. Violation of this confidentiality, even for the most humane of reasons, places the physician at legal risk. Informed consent refers to a patient's knowledgeable agreement to undergo a medical procedure.

471. The answer is C. *(Isselbacher, 13/e, pp 357–361.)* Several disorders have recently been found to be the result of expanding series of triplet repeats. These include the fragile X syndrome, myotonic dystrophy and Huntington's disease. Although the length of the region is variable in normal individuals, unaffected female carriers, and nonpenetrant, transmitting males have "premutations," which are generally 50 to 230 repeats in length. Individuals with premutations are, therefore, phenotypically unaffected. Nonpenetrant males transmit only unstable premutations; female carriers may transmit either premutations or full mutations, which are associated with mental retardation and the other phenotypic features of the syndrome.

472. The answer is D. *(Thompson, 5/e, p 391.)* This child has several minor anomalies, a major anomaly that affects the genitalia, and developmental delay. These multiply affected and embryologically unrelated body regions suggest a syndrome rather than a sequence. Because of the multiple anomalies and developmental delay, the first diagnostic test to be considered is a karyotype rather than a test for specific organ function, such as serum testosterone.

473. The answer is C. *(Thompson, 5/e, pp 92–94.)* The hypothetical probe D15S8 would imply a unique DNA segment that recognizes a single locus on chromosome 15—the eighth such anonymous DNA probe to be isolated. Since normal individuals have two number 15 chromosomes, they should have two alleles visualized after DNA restriction and hybridization with probe D15S8. Since both parents are heterozygous for the D15S8 locus as shown in part A of the figure that accompanies the question, the child's result suggests that he has only received the maternal alleles (alleles 1,2) for locus D15S8. This implies that he has received both number 15 chromosomes from his mother. This is known as *uniparental disomy* and may occur by correction of trisomy 15 conceptions through loss of the paternal number 15 chromosome.

474. The answer is D. *(Thompson, 5/e, pp 129–132.)* DNA fingerprinting is used in both paternity and forensic analyses and relies on highly variable DNA polymorphisms called variable numbers of tandem repeats (VNTRs). The multicopy repeats include $(CA)_n$ and minisatellite sequences that are present throughout the genome. The usual VNTR probe is directed against single-copy DNA that flanks these repeats and yields multiple restriction fragment sizes that reflect the number of intervening repeats. The hypothetical probes D7Z5 and D20Z1 shown in part B of the figure that accompanies the question recognize VNTR loci on chromosomes 7 and 20 that yield at least three alleles. Since the child's two alleles for D7Z5 (and D20Z1) match those of the mother and father, correct maternity and paternity are established with a degree of error equal to the chance that these allele combinations would occur in an unrelated individual. In practice, at least five VNTR probes are employed so that the odds for paternity (or nonpaternity) are very high indeed.

475. The answer is C. *(Thompson, 5/e, p 395.)* Informed consent requires that the patient be informed of all adverse effects that might result from a procedure. Evidence for nonpaternity may result from various types of DNA analysis and should be discussed with the concerned parties at the time of blood collection. Some physicians speak to the mother and father separately about this issue to maximize the opportunity for independent decision-making.

476. The answer is B. *(Thompson, 5/e, pp 92–94.)* Since the parents are heterozygous for differently sized D15S8 restriction fragment alleles, each allele becomes a marker for the respective parental 15 chromosome. The presence of alleles 1 and 2 in the child implies uniparental disomy with both maternal 15 chromosomes being passed to the child. This would represent heterodisomy, with both of the mother's number 15 chromosomes being passed down, as opposed to isodisomy where two copies of one maternal chromosome are transmitted. Uniparental isodisomy would make the child homozygous for a single restriction fragment allele and could not be distinguished from monosomy unless dosage or cytogenetic studies were performed. The presence of three chromosome 15 alleles would imply trisomy for the number 15 chromosome, and the particular parental alleles inherited would reveal the origin of the nondisjunction.

477. The answer is B. *(Thompson, 5/e, pp 92–94).* In humans and other mammals, the source of genetic material may be as important as its content.

Mice manipulated to receive two male pronuclei develop as abortive placentas, while those receiving two female pronuclei develop as abortive fetuses. The different impact of the same genetic material according to whether it is transmitted from mother or father is due to genomic imprinting. The term *imprinting* is borrowed from animal behavior and refers to parental marking during gametogenesis—the physical basis may be DNA methylation or chromatin phasing. Both maternally derived and paternally derived haploid chromosome sets are, thus, necessary for normal fetal development—this is why parthenogenesis does not occur in mammals. The imprint is erased in the fetal gonads and reestablished based on fetal sex. Certain cases of Prader-Willi syndrome are disorders of imprinting with the absence of the paternally imprinted chromosome 15.

478. The answer is E. *(Gelehrter, pp 255–262. Thompson, 5/e, pp 53–94.)* The isolated or sporadic case is a problem in genetic counseling because the pedigree is not helpful in determining recurrence risk. New mutations for autosomal or X-linked dominant disorders, new chromosomal rearrangements, autosomal recessive conditions, and nongenetic disorders may all present as the first case in a family. A negative family history does rule out multigenerational disease.

479. The answer is A. *(Gelehrter, pp 165–171. Thompson, 5/e, pp 207–208.)* The *arrow* in the figure points to the deletion of region 15q11q13 in one of the patient's number 15 chromosomes. This interstitial deletion is seen in approximately 50 percent of patients with Prader-Willi and Angelman syndromes. It is now known that imprinting of the 15q11q13 region is important in the genesis of these two syndromes.

480. The answer is C. *(Thompson, 5/e, pp 92–94.)* The presence of two chromosomes 15 in the partial karyotype excludes monosomy 15 as an answer. Paternal isodisomy is a possible answer, but paternal heterodisomy would require the presence of alleles 3 and 4. Presence of the D15S8 locus within the 15q13q15 deleted region is most likely based on the cytogenetic result; this implies that the maternal chromosome 15 was deleted since neither maternal allele is transmitted to the child.

481. The answer is B. *(Thompson, 5/e, pp 92–94.)* Since approximately 50 percent of patients with Prader-Willi or Angelman syndrome have identical deletions of 15q13q15, deletion alone cannot explain the differences between these syndromes. DNA probe analysis similar to that shown in the figure at question 473 has shown that the absence of 15q13q15 is on the maternally derived chromosome in Angelman syndrome and on the paternally derived chromosome in Prader-Willi syndrome. Uniparental disomy 15 from the mother would be equivalent to deleting the paternally imprinted 15q13q15 region and is found in Prader-Willi syndrome. Paternal uniparental disomy 15, though rare, has been demonstrated in Angelman syndrome.

482. The answer is C. *(Gelehrter, pp 179–189. Thompson, 5/e, pp 243–245.)* A peripheral blood karyotype provides the most reliable examination of the sex chromosomes. A bone marrow karyotype is more rapid (it uses rapidly dividing bone marrow cells) but usually has less resolution for defining subtle X and Y chromosome rearrangements. A buccal smear would theoretically show one Barr body in females (representing inactivation of one X chromosome) and none in males. In practice, this test is not very reliable and is rarely used. Detection of material of the Y long arm by polymerase chain reaction (PCR) would be useful but does not examine the Y short arm that contains the sex-determining region.

483. The answer is A. *(Gelehrter, pp 82–85, 171–176. Thompson, 5/e, pp 108–109, 243–245.)* The dot-blot demonstrates hybridization of the proband's DNA with the DXS14 and SRY DNA probes and establishes the diagnosis of a genetic male. Gender assignment is not based solely on genetic testing but must include surgical and reproductive prognoses for male versus female adult function. For these reasons, the patient with ambiguous genitalia is a medical emergency that requires delicate management until gender assignment is agreed upon. The proband, for example, was judged not to have adequate phallic tissue for reconstruction of normal male genitalia and underwent appropriate surgery for female gender assignment.

484. The answer is B. *(Gelehrter, pp 179–189. Thompson, 5/e, pp 243–245.)* True hermaphroditism implies the presence of both male and female genitalia in the same patient and is extremely rare. Male pseudohermaphroditism implies a genetic male with incomplete development of his genitalia, as in the proband. Causes can range from abnormalities of the pituitary-adrenal-gonadal hormone axis to local defects in tissue reponsiveness to testosterone. The XY female and XX male refer to phenotypically normal individuals whose genetic sex does not match their phenotypic sex. Examples include testicular feminization and pure gonadal dysgenesis (XY females) and offspring of fathers with Y translocations that inherit a cryptic SRY region without a visible Y chromosome (XX males).

485. The answer is B. *(Gelehrter, pp 171–176. Thompson, 5/e, p 391.)* Nondisclosure is generally inappropriate for a physician-patient relationship unless certain facts are judged to violate the higher doctrine of causing the patient no harm. Nondisclosure is more frequently used as a manner of presentation than as a withholding of facts—for example, by using terms such as "developmental delay" or "seriously ill" rather than emotionally charged terms such as "mental retardation" or "dying." In this case, the patient's necessary management as a female was considered most relevant for the parents so that her gender identity rather than genetic sex was stressed. Continuity of care is essential under such circumstances so that future medical problems can be appropriately managed.

486. The answer is A. *(Nelson, 2/e, pp 164–169.)* In the neonate, nonspecific symptoms such as poor feeding, lethargy, vomiting, respiratory distress, coma, and seizures may be signs of a multitude of disorders, including sepsis; diseases of the cardiopulmonary, gastrointestinal, and central nervous systems; and inborn errors of metabolism. A syndrome is a pattern of major and minor malformations and is not described in this infant.

487. The answer is E. *(Nelson, 2/e, pp 164–169.)* Since most inborn errors of metabolism are recessive disorders, parental consanguinity or a history of neonatal deaths within the same sibship are important clues. In addition, because a few inborn errors of metabolism are X-linked, it is also important to ask about neonatal deaths on the mother's side of the family. Since inborn errors of metabolism may involve an inability to metabolize various components of food, such as protein or fats, dietary history is extremely important. Several inborn errors also produce an unusual odor of the urine or sweat. Because inborn errors are single gene defects, a karyotype is not usually helpful in making the diagnosis.

488. The answer is B. *(Scriver, 6/e, pp 2083–2103.)* Most inborn errors of metabolism are inherited as autosomal recessive disorders. A family history of consanguinity would also suggest an autosomal recessive mode of inheritance.

489. The answer is B. *(Nelson, 2/e, pp 164–168.)* In treating inborn errors of metabolism that present acutely in the newborn period, aggressive fluid and electrolyte therapy and caloric supplementation are important to correct the imbalances caused by the disorder. Since many of the metabolites that build up in inborn errors of metabolism are toxic to the central nervous system, hemodialysis is recommended for any patient in stage II coma (poor muscle tone, few spontaneous movements, responsive to painful stimuli) or worse. Hemodialysis is 10 times as effective as peritoneal dialysis in removing toxic metabolites. Dietary therapy should minimize substances that cannot be metabolized—in this case valine, methionine, and isoleucine. Antibiotics are frequently useful since metabolically compromised children are more susceptible to infection.

490. The answer is B. *(Gelehrter, pp 32–36.)* In this example, mutations in different genes and at different loci can produce a similar phenotype. This phenomenon is known as *genetic heterogeneity.* In *allelic heterogeneity,* different mutations at the same locus may produce abnormal phenotypes. *Penetrance* is the all-or-none expression of the gene, while *expressivity* refers to the variation in the degree of severity of the phenotype. *Dosage compensation* is a phenomenon related to X-inactivation.

491. The answer is C. *(Gelehrter, pp 202–207. Thompson, 5/e, pp 178–190.)* The recurrence risk for an autosomal recessive disorder is 1 in 4, or 25 percent.

492. The answer is C. *(Gelehrter, pp 202–207. Thompson, 5/e, pp 178–190.)* The proband in this case has inherited the A allele from one parent and the B allele from the other. However, it is impossible to determine which allele came from which parent. The fetus has the same genotype as his affected brother. However, it cannot be determined if he inherited these alleles from the same parents as the affected boy and is, thus, affected or from the opposite parents and, thus, is an unaffected noncarrier. It can be said that he is definitely not an unaffected carrier. Assuming no recombination has occurred, the risk for the fetus to be affected is 1/2, or 50 percent.

493–495. The answers are: 493-B, 494-E, 495-D. *(Gelehrter, pp 125–157. Thompson, 5/e, pp 276–282.)* Metabolic diseases always exhibit autosomal or X-linked recessive inheritance. Autosomal recessive inheritance is most likely in view of the parental consanguinity and the affected sisters. Regardless of their consanguinity, the proband's parents are obligate carriers and will have a 1/4 chance to have a fourth affected child. (Remember that chance has no memory, so the prior affected siblings do not affect the recurrence risk.) The normal sibling has a 2/3 chance of being a carrier, a 1/4 chance that her cousin is also a carrier, and a 1/4 chance of having an affected child given the first two conditions. If she marries her cousin, the risk is $2/3 \times 1/4 \times 1/4 = 1/24$ of having an affected child. If she marries an unrelated man, his chance to be a carrier is $2pq$ from the Hardy-Weinberg equilibrium. Since the incidence of Hurler syndrome (given as 1/10,000 but actually 5 or 10-fold lower) is q^2, $q = 1/100$ and $2pq$, then the incidence of carriers is 1/50. The final risk for the unrelated couple is 2/3 × 1/50 × 1/4 = 1/300.

496. The answer is D. *(Thompson, 5/e, pp 278–282.)* The introduction of two different genetic mutations into a cell or organism to see if they correct one another is called a complementation test. Successful complementation means that the deficiencies in each cell line must effect different genetic loci (i.e., genetic rather than allelic heterogeneity). If cell fusion is used, as with somatic cell hybridization, then the gene products from each loci are present in the same cell. In the case of the mucopolysaccharidoses, cell cultures from different patients were inadvertently mixed and, in some cases, found to correct each other. Since the cells were not fused, correction required targeting of an enzyme from one type of cell to the lysosomes of another. This mechanism was later shown to involve mannose-6-phosphate groups attached to the enzyme.

497. The answer is A. *(Gelehrter, pp 283–286. Thompson, 5/e, pp 317–336.)* Enzyme therapy (i.e., injection of purified enzyme) has been successful in several lysosomal deficiencies, particularly those in which the central nervous system is unaffected (i.e., Gaucher's disease). Unfortunately, antibodies frequently develop that limit successful enzyme delivery. Somatic gene therapy (i.e., delivery of enzyme to somatic cells via viral vectors or transfected tissue) is now possible; however, targeting of the gene product to appropriate tissues and organelles is still a problem. Transfected autologous bone marrow transplant (i.e., marrow from the patient) has worked well in adenosine deaminase deficiency, an immune disorder affecting lymphocytes. Germ-line gene therapy requires the insertion of functional genes into gametes or blastomeres of early embryos *prior* to birth. The potential for embryonic damage, lack of knowledge regarding developmental gene control, and ethical controversies regarding selective breeding or embryo experimentation make germ-line therapy unrealistic at present.

498. The answer is C. *(Thompson, 5/e, pp 337–347.)* The probability that any one sibling is homozygous normal is 1/3. The human leukocyte antigen (HLA) cluster on chromosome 6 consists of several loci that are each highly polymorphic. Because the loci are clustered together, their polymorphic products form haplotypes (i.e., A1-B8-DR2 on one chromosome and A9-B5-DR3 on another chromosome). Since recombination among HLA loci is unlikely, the chances for two siblings to be HLA identical is essentially that of inheriting the same parental chromosomes, that is, 1/4. For a sibling to be both homozygous normal for Hurler syndrome and HLA compatible, the chance is

$1/3 \times 1/4 = 1/12$. Since there are three siblings, the total chance is $1/12 \times 3$, or $1/4$.

499. The answer is E. *(Gelehrter, pp 171–176. Thompson, 5/e, pp 411–425.)* The physician is obligated to describe a patient's disease accurately in the medical record and to share such records with legally entitled entities such as health insurance companies. Although care should be exercised that records containing confidential information are not shared inappropriately, there was no such breach of confidentiality in this case. If the physician had declined further care without appropriate notice, then this would be a breach of ongoing care. However, insurance companies and managed care plans have excluded patients because of prior conditions or excessive expenses (i.e., capitation limits). This does constitute discrimination, but application of the American Disabilities Act to patients with genetic diseases is not yet routine. These dilemmas will grow dramatically with the increasing ability to test for genetic diseases and predispositions.

500. The answer is D. *(Gelehrter, pp 275–283. Thompson, 5/e, pp 411–425.)* Most enzymes are expressed in chorionic villi or amniocytes and allow prenatal diagnosis of metabolic disorders through cell culture and enzyme assay. Percutaneous umbilical blood sampling (PUBS), or cordocentesis, offers another strategy if the enzyme is normally present in leukocytes. Alpha-fetoprotein (AFP) is not known to be involved in any metabolic disorders, but it is used as an index of fetal tissue differentiation and integrity. Maternal serum α-fetoprotein (MSAFP) would not be useful in a case of normal fetal development with L-iduronidase deficiency.

Bibliography

Gelehrter TD, Collins FS: *Principles of Medical Genetics.* Baltimore, Williams & Wilkins, 1990.

Isselbacher KJ, Braunwald E, Wilson JD, Martin JB, Fauci AS, Kasper DL (eds): *Harrison's Principles of Internal Medicine,* 13/e. New York, McGraw-Hill, 1994.

McKusick VA: *Mendelian Inheritance in Man.* Baltimore, Johns Hopkins University Press, 1992.

Nelson NM: *Current Therapy in Neonatal-Perinatal Medicine,* 2/e. Philadelphia, BC Decker, 1989.

Scriver CR, Beaudet AL, Sly WS, Valle D: *The Metabolic Basis of Inherited Disease,* 6/e. New York, McGraw-Hill, 1989.

Thompson MW, McInnes RR, Willard HF: *Genetics in Medicine,* 5/e. Philadelphia, WB Saunders, 1991.